Bioenergy Body Balance

A Guide to Healthy Living

Dr. Miriam Thomas Keele

Self Published

ISBN 978-3-033-03701-4 -- Paperback Book
ISBN 978-3-033-04126-4 -- Electronic Book

Cover Design: Rosmarie Iadarola
Editing: James Keele

Please visit us also at:
http://www.bioenergy-balance.com
http://bioenergieheilung.ch

Notice:
This book is intended as a reference source only, not as a substitute for medical advice. The information given here is designed to help you make informed decisions about your health. It is not intended as a substitute for any treatment that may have been prescribed by your doctor. If you suspect that you have a medical problem, we urge you to seek competent medical help.

DEDICATION

This book is dedicated to my husband
James for his love
and for bringing light into my life

and

to my son Vedran
who gave my life a meaning

PREFACE OF THE AUTHOR

This book was created as the result of my knowledge and studies of Holistic medicine for my own needs as well as by working with my patients.

Always having had an insight in the newest scientific studies, I realised that there is an ugent need for necessary and accurate information, and corresponding assistance found in one place. This brought me to a decision to gather the information all into one place and write down everything that one person can do to help to preserve hers or his health. I was led by my own needs, but also very often by the despair that I saw in the eyes of my patients on their yearning for help.

Twenty years ago dealing with my medical profession, I noticed a need to know more, and I started with further training in the fields of holistic medicine. The road was long, and brought me to my intensive involvement and immersion in the area of therapy with clinical medical hypnosis, which I am practicing today together with bioenergy therapy. In this way I am helping my patients and sharing my knowledge of Psychoneuroimmunology with the students of the Holistic Academy. On my way to gather knowledge in holistic medicine, I have come to believe that holistic medicine as well as Psychoneuroimmunology combined with the knowledge of school medicine and holistic medicine fused together in a complementary science, provide the greatest impact and contribution to my patients, family and to me personally.

Dr. Miriam Thomas Keele
Schwyz
Switzerland

For further questions about therapies and courses you can contact me at these Web sites:

http://www.bioenergy-balance.com
http://bioenergieheilung.ch
http://hypnosetherapie-schweiz.com

THANKS

Hereby I want to thank all those who have encouraged me in so many different ways, and have helped me so that this book could become a reality.

I am grateful to my husband James, whose expertise in the field of computer science, programming and editing helped immensely.

Furthermore, I would like to thank my assistent and secretary Milijana Savic, for her dedication, skills and loyalty by performing all the tasks entrusted to her, and for her support while working on this book.

I thank my partners in the field of Hypnosis Therapy, Rudolf Corcchia and Katja Berini, for the knowledge and skills that they shared with me. Last but not least I would like to thank my graphic designer, Rosmarie Iadarola, for the graphic layout of the cover.

Table of Contents

Introduction 13

Chapter 1 - A Guide for Living 17

Chapter 2 - Overblown Myths and Dogmas 28

Chapter 3 - Bioenergy 49

Chapter 4 - Electromagnetic Waves 53

Electromagnetic Waves
Brain Waves
Bioenergy and Scalar Waves

Chapter 5 - The Application of Scalar Waves 67

Lightning Balls of Nikola Tesla
Philadelphia Experiment
Project HAARP
Positive use of bioenergy
The God's Code
The Field of Positive Intentions
The Development and Recent History of Bioenergy Treatments
Healing with Bioenergy

Chapter 6 - Bioenergetic Medicine 86

The Levels of a Human Being
Physical Health and Diseased Conditions
Aura
Yin and Yang
Chakras
Immune System
Self-Control of the Mind and How to Achieve
the Field of Positive Intention
Types of Meditation and Contemplative
Neuroscience
How to Change Yourself

Chapter 7 - Bioenergy Therapies 126

What is Bioenergy Therapy?
How Is Bioenergy Therapy Performed?
Medical Hypnosis Therapy
Application of Clinical Medical Hypnosis in
Psychoneuroimmunology
Jin Shin Jyutsu
Thai Yoga Therapy
Ayurveda

Chapter 8 – Holistic Sports 178

Tai Chi
Pilates

Chapter 9 – Nutrition 196

Vegetarianism
Veganism
Pros and Cons About Vegetarianism and
Traps of Vegetarianism

Chapter 10 – Dietetics 205

Natural substitutes and dietary supplements
Vitamins as Natural Supplements
Minerals as Natural Supplements
Coenzyme Q 10
L Glutamine
Omega-3 Fatty Acids
Enzymes
Enzyme in the Battle Against Cancer

Chapter 11 - When, How, Why and What To Eat 239

Metabolic Types of People
Vata Dosha
Pitta Dosha
Kapha Dosha
The Effect of Cortisol
Metabolic Syndrome
Circadian Rhythm, or Circadian Biological Clock

Chapter 12 - Bioenergy and food 275

Chapter 13 - Bioenergy Body Balance Diet – BBB Diet 277

The Basics of the BBB Diet
Who can benefit from the BBB Diet
The BBB Diet Guidelines
Getting ready for the Bioenergy Body Balance Diet
Protocol of the Bioenergy Body Balance Diet

Chapter 14 – Recipes 315

Links 326

References 327

Introduction

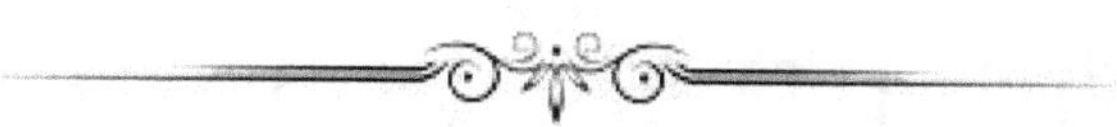

Never before has mankind had more opportunities to live in accordance with his wish for longevity, knowing that the development of medicine only in the last two decades has opened the way to a better, higher quality and longer life of the human race.

The average age of people in America during the 1950's, during the last century, was only 52 years of age. Today, sixty years later, the average age has increased to 70 years of age. What makes someone really aware of huge progress is that we are talking about averages; people over age of 90, including centenarians, are no longer a rarity.

Is it enough and do we have to stop by that level? Certainly not.

There are still many fields of medicine that are frenetically searching for urgent answers. Scientists all over the world are desperately looking and racing to find a treatment for numerous diseases that are not treatable at the moment. A whole army of desperate people harmed by incurable diseases, are waiting to be cured.

Is there any chance that this is going to happen in the foreseeable future? This question can be surely answered with a clear yes. Is there any time frame to predict when this will happen? It is happening right now and here. It has been among us for centuries. But awareness about these treatments, like many things in the life of a human being, is a kind of process that has been suppressed and is now developing slowly. The idea of Bioenergy medicine and related healing methods has been roughly known and spread all over the world. Very few people know what the variety of methods and principles of Bioenergy really are.

The process has been basically developed within two groups of people, regardless of their education. The people that were interested in nature and tradition, which exists in every nation in the world, had a feeling of being connected with nature. Among them were many physicians. They were open for new knowledge and were curious enough to initiate their path of education in all kind of natural medicine branches. The other group created itself out of those who did not find the help they suddenly and many times urgently needed in a conventional school of medicine.

This "School Medicine" is named that way because it is taught at the high universities in the world very profoundly and comprehensively about structure, function, dysfunction and treatment of the human body. And at the same time, it is called "conventional" because it acknowledges empirical knowledge. This simply means that all of the statements and claims have to be proven in order to become medically approved, and applied on human beings.

All other branches of medicine which trace their roots over thousands of years in the past, transferring their knowledge from generation to generation are classified in a common group called "Alternative Medicine". Some of the results of this method are provable, and some of them are not. But all of them, despite of significant progress in the last 20 years, are put in this common group called "Alternative Medicine". This is completely a wrong category and name to start with, because the methods, techniques and treatments are crossing each other and complimenting each other, no matter if they are coming from school medicine or traditional natural medicine. Therefore, we can and have to speak only about "Complimentary Medicine".

Bioenergy medicine is one such of these complimentary branches. In this book I am going to reveal to you how you can help, in the first place, yourself, as well as your family and people that are close to you. I will also help you to achieve something that should be the most important thing in the world to you - to stay or become healthy, happy, attractive and successful. And at the same time look at least 10 years younger.

My knowledge will be described as well as the methods that I use on myself and am teaching, in order to protect you from most of the illnesses, physical and mental, and give you a general feeling of well being, associated with a motivation towards creativity and success.

You will be taught, from my own personal experiences, how to fight and come to the final goal of staying healthy without reaching for medications for every little imbalance you might have. Especially not those groups of medications that are causing you more harm than good. I am going to teach you how to change your life for your own favor and benefit, and how to become fit, well shaped, and filled with energy. I will show you how to do everything possible to protect your body, mind and spirit from disease and bad environmental influences, which includes your own self. This will include showing you the causes that lead to disease and how to bring everything into a balance, Bioenergy Body Balance.

This is at the same time the sense of Holistic Medicine. It is regarding the human being as a unity of body, mind and spirit connected with the universe.

Chapter 1

A Guide for Living

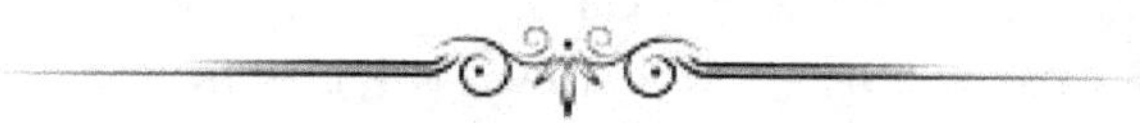

1. Try not to dwell constantly with thoughts about yourself, your problems or your fears.

If we constantly keep thinking about what is going on in and around us, we become very sensitive for every little detail. Then we are "blowing up" with no need, creating unneeded anxiety, and making a "mountain out of a molehill". We even go further and ingrain thoughts within our minds and start fearing the things that are not going to happen in the future.

2. Try to start enjoying your profession or the work that you are performing.

The one that hates his job or profession repeatedly experiences increased pressure and stress every day. This increase in pressure and stress on a daily basis leads certainly to physical dysfunction or disease.

3. Find any kind of activity that makes you feel good, and creates a feeling of joy within yourself.

Such activity is helping us to relax during our free time

and is helping us to enjoy the activities that please and entertain us. Thinking of such activities while we are working will make us feel good within one second by imagining how we are going to enjoy our time off or weekend. By doing so, we will perform our work easier, faster and with less effort.

4. Try to start sympathizing, or at least accepting, the people around you.

Let's face it. There are people that you do not enjoy associating with. However, we cannot completely avoid their coexistence. There are people that we have to meet on a daily basis, whether we like it or not. It is unavoidable. So let's try to look for and find their good side – every human being has his good qualities and merits. It is up to you to take the time to look for them – for your own sake and benefit – because everything is relative.

5. Try to accept the circumstances that you cannot change.

Personal Creed – " Grant me the serenity to accept the thing I cannot change, the courage to change the things I can, and the wisdom to know the difference."

Circumstances that we cannot change are, for each of us, a fact and the reality of our lives. A person that is constantly upset by the circumstances in his own life is constantly very angry and upset. It even goes so far that he starts hating his own life and environment. This person is not only an indigestible person, but he is certainly going to get sick on a physical level, sooner or later.

6. Never allow life situations to prevail over you.

Each of us who gives in, hangs down his head and is being suppressed by such situations is prone to psychosomatic diseases. This defeat will not leave us in peace. As the result, damages will show within time in your physical body and will force us to deal with larger problems than that which we had before.

7. Be kind to the people around you.

Instead of making some mean or vicious comments that come upon our mind, we should rather keep silent, and not say anything. My mother always taught me that if we cannot say something nice, say nothing at all. We should use the first opportunity to express a kind word or a complement to our partner, friend, coworker or any other person.

Try it right away, and your life will become much more pleasant for both parties.

8. Be resolute, reasonable and keep your common sense.

It is absolutely inappropriate to close your eyes in front of the facts, and to fool yourself.

Hoping that things will be solved somehow in the future and work out in your favor, despite of the difficulties that are piling up in front of you, and putting your head in the sand like an ostrich, is unrealistic and damaging.

So let me tell you - this is not going to happen.

Sooner or later, we will have to face the difficulties and the facts the way they are. The sooner that we tidy up our matters, do what we need to do, the issue that we have is going to diminish and, at the end, we will get rid of it. If you are in any kind of difficulty and whatever your difficulty might be, always keep in mind that the success to solve your difficulty is depending upon your approach. You should by all means take care that you do not suffer in your own suffering. If you meet a person that is more knowledgeable than you are, pay careful attention to what this person is saying and try to learn as much as you can.

Whatever it is that you are doing, or what might be a matter of your interest, pay significant attention to the details. The details are a tiny part of the whole from which everything depends.

9. Never waste your life on unimportant matters.

It can happen to us very easily that we do not see the tree for the forest.

10. Do not over exaggerate in anything that you do.

No matter how big is your bank account.

11. Stop smoking.

Stop smoking if you are a constant smoker over the entire day, especially, if smoking is not a pleasurable habit in your leisure time. There are a few options to stop smoking, and I will share them with you.

12. Alcohol consumption.

Consume alcohol only occasionally and never on a regular basis. If you prefer wine, one glass of red wine in the evening will not harm you.

13. Food consumption.

Eat foods according to your needs, knowledge and ability to find the right kind of food. You should find the proper types of food, i.e. organic. You can find an organic food store, or even search for the local farmers market.

Last but not least, close the kitchen after 8 o'clock in the evening.

Try to never eat processed foods, i.e. canned foods and pre-cooked foods, which is one of the most difficult tasks. If you think of it in detail, you will realize that I am right, and nowadays it is very difficult because everything is processed.

This way your vital organs and your body, specifically your immune system, will stay healthy and be able to defend itself against disease. At the same time, you will become slim, and full of energy. You will amaze yourself and the other people around you and your intervals of sickness will become shorter in duration and intensity. Most importantly, you will impede inflammation in your body that is leading to diseases of the vital organs, aging of the body, and death.

A human being that is always healthy and does not get sick does not exist. If someone is telling you this, they might be pulling your leg.

But if some of the facts regarding dieting offered here will meet your biological needs, you should choose the ones that will meet your biological rhythm, taste, and your purchasing ability, in order to create your own menu. This way you can feed yourself and your family with healthy foods of your own choice.

Most importantly, you will not consume foods just by chance. You will understand what exactly you are eating. You will know the reasons why some foods should always be consumed, some foods occasionally, and some foods never.

Make two different daily meal plans, each for a seven-day period, and then change them every week. Keep a third list of foods that you can add or replace in any one of the meal plans. This way you do not need to beat yourself up about what you are going to eat, and spend considerable time and effort to get quality nutrition. It is not necessary to constantly reinvent the recipes, digging through them. Some recipes include preparation for twenty ingredients or more. This might cause you to get tired of everything and return to your old habits.

14. Annual Doctor Checkups.

Lay down this book immediately, grab your phone and arrange for an appointment for a blood test and blood pressure measurements.

Diagnostics have made the greatest progress in today's medicine with no doubt. Before you can start working on yourself, you must know the status of your health. Your diet as well as your choice of physical activity depends upon the status of your health. If possible make a test for food intolerance. This test is very important because it will show you which foods you are not digesting well, and which foods are to be avoided. In addition, the test is an indicator of your metabolism, and is valid only for you. Food intolerance is a very dangerous thing. It sneaks into the body slowly and without the person being aware of it and is a real life "body snatcher". The food that is being partially digested is poisoning you from the inside. Since you are not allergic to this food, you have no allergic reaction that would otherwise make you aware of the fact that you are having a problem and that you have to avoid those foods. Chronic inflammation is slowly created throughout your body without your being aware of it, and this is a life-threatening situation.

15. Review the medications that you take.

Medications taken randomly, on an irregular basis or because you are "your own doctor" could be poisoning you.

Review with your doctor the type and amount of medications you are taking. Do not change anything on your own. Do not stop taking prescribed medications.

16. Do not try to change the people around you.

You are losing your time, energy and effort if you think you will succeed in changing someone else. Since you cannot succeed in that, you are becoming frustrated and are as a matter of fact inducing stress, which will lead you into a disease.

Instead, try to change yourself. Because the only person you can change is you.

17. Start a regular physical program activity of your choice on a daily or weekly basis.

What you are going to choose for an activity depends on your affiliations that are different for each person. Never forget: we are all different. There are physical activities that you can practice alone, or those that are performed in groups. No matter what you decide, make sure that you are going to do your best to defend and promote your mental, spiritual, and the physical state of your body, allowing constant and uninterrupted flow of your bioenergy. And that is the only guarantee of preserving your health.

18. The biggest burden that you have to overcome is you.

Force yourself to control your thoughts. Do this every day on a regular basis. The person that succeeds in controlling his thoughts and bringing them to a higher level is improving and changing his whole body.

In this book, you will find the methods that will help you to succeed in this on your own. Of course, if you are having any serious problem that would need to be assisted by a professional, you should do so.

Today there are a large number of different methods and treatments of all types. They will not all be listed here. I will talk only about those which I have tested on myself personally, and which I am still using. That way I am helping my family, my friends, my patients, and myself.

19. Defend the wellbeing of your vegetative nervous system by all means.

This means that we should get plenty of sleep, keep a well scheduled and routine lifestyle, take regular vacations, spend a certain amount of time in outdoor activities with fresh air, physical exercise and mental hygiene in dedicated timeframes, eat healthy and try to spend your time off pleasantly. Doing so, we can reach the bioenergy balance in our body, mind and soul, and we will become healthy and stay healthy for a long period of time.

20. Understand and accept that within each of us both good and evil is contained.

It is depending on us to try by all means to keep our balance and acquire skills that will keep our evil under control. It is only in this way that we will enable our intelligent energy, which exists all-around us, to flow smoothly and without hindrance through our body. This will enable this intelligent energy to influence the body and initiate the self-healing process that your body requires, allowing the bioenergy of our body, mind and spirit to be in harmony and balance. Bioenergy Body Balance.

Chapter 2

Overblown Myths and Dogmas

We all know the definition of a myth. It is when facts about someone or something that is deeply cut into the human consciousness become law, whether it is written or unwritten. Myths are unbeatable, historical, factual and eternal. However, this is a new time. The myths and dogmas in medicine are beginning to fall because scientific studies have proven that some previous beliefs are inaccurate. It has happened from time to time in human history that a myth would turn out to be wrong, but it is more prevalent now since these are very vibrant times, full of action, changes, and reciprocities. New research is occurring daily, proving as many times in the past that some firm beliefs are turning out to be wrong. But are these beliefs wrong? Well at least it should make us think very sharply about it.

Why do we tend to believe so strongly in something? There is a psychological study by Mr. Gary Taubes who states that within our consciousness exists a condition called "cognitive dissidence." When you, for instance, become aware that you have been making the wrong assumptions all of your working life about a certain matter, your brain will, in that case, find a way to convince you that you have always been right. This is one of the mechanisms that hold the dogmas firmly bonded in their positions for a very long time.

Let me tell you of some of the myths or dogmas that have been proven incorrect or wrong by the latest scientific evidence.

1. Salt

There is a premise that salt causes high blood pressure, and has become a myth. This is, in fact, only partially correct based on the newest research from the scientific point of view. A very significant number of individuals are having an increased blood pressure when the salt intake is higher, but it has been proven that this does not affect everyone in the same manner. There are many people who consume salt, but do not develop high blood pressure.

Do not start to make plans on salting your meals from now on because you believe someone has given you herewith a "green light" to do so. So do not start consuming salt like a goat.

No human body is the same. Call for an appointment with your doctor and check the condition of the status of your organs. It is not yet clear why some people have no problems, let alone damages, by consuming salt and some do. Also it has been determined that all edible salts are not the same. One type will clog the vessels, while other types have beneficial effects on the body and have definite healing qualities.

Common *edible table salt* consists of approximately 97.5% sodium chloride and 2.5% of other chemicals such as iodine and moisture absorbents. It is dried in processing at 1,200 ° F. This high heat alters the natural chemical structure of the salt.

Ordinary table salt, which can cause damage to health, has nothing in common with *unrefined natural salt*, which is an essential ingredient for proper biological function of the body. However, if your health condition can allow greater consumption of salt, keep in mind that you need to have a balance between sodium and potassium. Potassium weakens the impact of Sodium on raising the blood pressure. The latest studies are showing that already the daily dose of 1600 mg of potassium significantly reduces cases of stroke. That dose can be achieved by eating two bananas and one avocado a day. For a higher daily dose of, for example, 4700 mg per day, you can eat fish, spinach, natural yogurt and potatoes with the peels.

Consuming these foods is an individual choice and only those foods, which you are not hypersensitive to, should be included in your diet. More information on hypersensitivity to foods can be found in the chapter about nutrition.

For cooking and dieting use only natural unrefined sea salt.

In the markets and grocery stores of almost all countries, there is a fairly wide selection of salt products. Here are some:

- Himalayan salt - can be purchased in stores or organic food stores online
- Fleur de sel
- Natural Sea Salt
- Kosher Salt

2. Milk and dairy products

Milk and all dairy products have been considered to be a food necessity for the body for quite a while, and one of the main foundations of a healthy diet.

But this is not true for all people.

First and foremost, it is proven, that milk is not good for the digestion of adults, in difference to infants and young children.

Secondly, some people cannot consume milk or any product that contains milk, because they are confronted with serious digestive problems that are progressing if they do not discontinue eating dairy products.

This includes not only those people who are allergic to milk and dairy products, but it is also very significant for people who have intolerance to lactose. Allergy and lactose intolerance is the inability of the body to break down the process of digesting specific milk sugars. These sugars that many people are not able to digest are ending up in the intestines. Therefore they are causing an overgrowth of bacteria and fungi that are normally found in the intestinal flora. This is happening most commonly at the transition between the small to the large intestine. It is causing:

- Puffiness,
- Winds
- Cramps
- Diarrhea or constipation
- Depression
- Heartburn
- Fatigue
- Headaches

Lactose is a milk sugar and disaccharide. All kinds of milk, no matter if the origin is from cows, sheep or goats, contains lactose.

Besides these two groups of people, there are also people who have a variety of other types of allergies and/or hypersensitivities to these groups of food and they are also not supposed to consume milk and dairy products in general.

There are also people who are very allergic or simply not able to digest casein protein, which is a milk protein. Individuals can be allergic to milk sugar, of milk protein, or of both.
http://www.muscleandstrength.com/expert-guides/casein-protein

The consumption of milk is also absolutely not recommended to people who are prone to chronic sinus infections. Under the influence of milk, the mucosa of our sinus cavities will produce excessive mucus.

One of the most important things that must always be kept in mind is that everyone is different. We are all individuals but were created in a single mold.

Take time and the patience to find out which food is meeting your digestive needs in the best way, and which foods, on the other hand, are not good for your digestion.

If you are among those who do not consume milk and dairy products, remember it is not a reason to turn to processed foods and artificial products. One of the main rules with which you cannot go wrong is by choosing your foods that remain close to the soil as much as possible, i.e. local products, seasonal food, fresh food from the market, directly from the manufacturer, or from home grown plants in your garden, terrace or balcony.

3. Water

The latest scientific research that has been recently published by Australian scientists has confirmed that the myth that you have to drink ten glasses or about 2 liters of water a day is inaccurate.

Water is indispensable for life. Human beings have to maintain a balance of water in their bodies.

But to cover the need for water of a healthy person, more water does not mean ultimately a guarantee of better health. Exceptions are only the people in hot or dry climates, athletes and people with certain diseases. Those people have an increased need for intake of water.

People, who are practicing in the gym under normal thermal conditions or in an air-conditioned tennis hall, have no physiological need to fill themselves constantly with a liquid. Take a look when you are in the gym, on the tennis court or any other sport activity. You will see people that are having bottles with water or even isotonic liquids everywhere around them: on the gym machine, bike, body etc. Even elderly people have heard of it, so they decided to go with tradition and do something for their health. You can see people all around, pulling out their water bottles and drinking. It has been so aggressively pushed everywhere in the media, so that people have been brainwashed concerning water. You cannot even read about any of thousands of diet plans offered all around the world without being bombed with something like...be sure to drink at least 2 liters of water daily. Why exactly they are doing it and what is a balanced formula behind the amount of water that you should pour into yourself, whether you like it or not? They say that nobody knows for sure.

On the contrary, we do know. Our body has a built-in mechanism for the control of water balance - this is thirst.

Have you ever heard of the truth about water poisoning? Excessive consumption of water can result in a dangerous and life threatening toxic condition, which can end up to be fatal.

What has made us to believe that we should be pouring water into ourselves constantly? Aggressive marketing and the industry that produces bottled water are having their contribution on that. Not to speak about the variety of energy drinks that is a "must" to improve your physical prowess.

According to Dr. S. Goldfarb, specialist in urology, and Dr. D. Negoionu from the University of Pennsylvania in Philadelphia, there are 4 main myths about the intake of an excessive amount of water into the body, which "do not hold water":

- Flushing toxins from the body
- Enhancing skin tone
- Decreased feelings of hunger
- Reducing headaches

A normal physical body loses about 10 cups of water a day through sweating, urination, exhalation, and other normal bodily functions. By food consumption, we take in about 4 cups of liquid a day. In addition to that, one must add all the drinks that we are consuming during the day, regardless of whether those drinks are carbonated or not, caffeinated or not, or sweetened with sugars and artificial sweeteners. Everything that we drink goes into the total liquid intake, with the exception of alcohol. Alcohol is the only drink that doesn't bring water to the body, but is, in matter of fact, subtracting it out from the body.

One of the victims of water poisoning, respectively excessive intake of fluids into the body, was world-famous artist Andy Warhol, who died of a cardiac arrhythmia. His family sued the hospital because the death occurred as a direct result of excessive fluid intake in the patient's body through a drip causing hyper-hydration or water poisoning after a routine gallbladder operation.

Studies that have been carried out on the desert nomads have shown that people in very extreme conditions can fulfill the requirement of the body for water, with only a minimum water intake.

The Army has also made changes to the rules of fluid intake for its troops, which is needed for the human body and is sufficient but will not adversely affect their readiness.

On September 12, 1999, a soldier in the U.S. Air Force, M.J. Schindler, died of a heart attack two days after excessive intake of water during a routine military drill march of 5.8 miles. As a result, the U.S. Air Force has changed the requirements of the training of recruits.

People are equally dying of dehydration as well as of excessive intake of fluids in the body in a short time.

You should rely on your own need for liquid and only

drink when you feel thirst. Otherwise, avoid drinking liquids.

A reliable and easy way to evaluate this, according to Dr. D. Pierce, University Chief at McMaster University in Hamilton, Ontario, Canada, is the self-urine-control. If your urine is dark yellow, then you are on the right track, if it is very bright and clear, you need to drink less water.

4. Why many diets lead to failure

Myth of the calories

Many diets lead to failure because we eat the wrong foods (meaning the wrong composition of foods); we combine the wrong group of foods, are eating excessive portions or just eating at the wrong time of a day.

More about foods can be found in the chapter about nutrition.

For decades all kinds of possible and impossible diets, some of them I would even call bizarre, are appearing on the market. Many diets are created to eat only certain foods daily with the amount eaten not being important. The Atkins diet recommends that you eat meat (protein) and fat until you drop. Those who already have health problems are getting heart attacks and some even need urgent bypass operations. For some people who are sticking with the Atkins diet, there is no escape. There is a well-known case of a 20-year-old girl who died in 2001 due to the implementation of the Atkins diet. Such excessive amount of protein is a real shock to the kidneys, especially if the kidneys are, with a particular individual, the generally weaker organ. So you have people who are drastically dropping their weight and are reaching their desired weight. But on the other hand, this diet recommends a dangerous and aggressive intake of protein and fat with the possibility that can certainly lead to a catastrophic state of their body. It does not hurt to say that Atkins himself has died of a heart attack.

There are very many serious diets based on scientific research. One of them is a Low Glycemic Diet by Dr. David Jenkins from Toronto University. His diet has been created for the needs of people with diabetes or diabetes mellitus, and is based for this purpose on the Glycemic index (GI). GI is simply described as a number on a scale from 1 to 100 that indicates how many carbohydrates are contained in certain foods and are raising blood sugar levels. Of course, there is a "but", and this refers to the immense difference about which type of sugar is consumed. Thus, those people for whom it has been created in the first place - diabetics, should apply the diet.

You can learn more about that in my book about dieting, Bioenergy Body Balance (BBB) Diet.

In reality, thousands and thousands of mostly useless diets are published in the form of books, brochures, inside various magazines and all of them only created to increase sales and profits. This is, in particular, the case in the marketing campaigns for New Year's Resolutions. Many diet products are sold when people become determined to make a change for the better in their lives, to make up a decision to take their own lives in their own hands or to be able to wear that sexy bikini again for the next summer vacation. Well, at the end, many women still wear a two-piece swimsuit, but not a bikini. Instead they wear a tankini, because the diet was not a success.

A phrase that Dr. Robert Lustig emphasizes in dieting is: "Isocaloric but not isometabolic." What does that mean? It breaks the myth about all those impressive and potent diets that are preaching a variety of diverse abnormal conditions. Describing it simply, it means that you can consume the same amount of calories of glucose and fructose (fruit sugar and plain sugar), or fructose and protein, or fructose and fatty acids. But with each of these groups of foods that are basically having the same caloric value, you will establish a completely different metabolic memory of the body. These metabolic memories will hereafter be responsible for the chain of hormonal reactions, and these hormonal responses will be responsible for how much fat will accumulate in the body. To cut it short: it matters what kind of food you are consuming in the same meal. The food most responsible for the accumulation of the fat cells and obesity is fructose.

You can read more about that in the Chapter about food and dieting.

Exactly the same number of calories of different foods, or groups of foods, has a diametrically and dramatically different effect, despite the fact that the calories are calculated and carefully composed implying energetically conditions. No matter how you count the calories, it will not help you in losing weight if you are having the wrong combination of foods that are having the same number of calories. Now it does not mean that you can consume excessive amount of calories since you are not counting calories anymore, which is also a catch of many diets. The counting of calories has become a burden so many diets tell you not to count calories at all. This is partially true in that you do not need to count single calories, but should keep track of the total amount of calories. On the other hand, if you take the maximum number of calories as your daily limits, it significantly matters about the combination of the foods.

The only diets that are based on the laws of the metabolic functioning of the body will be listed in the Chapter about nutrition.

The total daily amount of calories that are consumed though cannot be ignored, but it has its own rules. By a certain weight, our body burns a certain number of calories. If your weight is decreased, meaning a conscious loss of weight, the number of calories that we are burning daily is lower. Our metabolism adapts to a specific number of calories that we constantly have to decrease if we want to lose more weight. Otherwise, we will reach a certain "Plateau", i.e., the limit at which the metabolism of the body adapts to the number of calories being consumed and we are not losing weight any more. To continue with weight loss, we must keep on decreasing the number of calories per day, but of course should not be under our basic needs.

Total daily caloric intake of less than 600 calories is considered insufficient, i.e., 600 calories is the lowest daily calorie intake limit, below which there is damage to the body and results in anorexia nervosa. At the same time, the plateau is a breaking point at which we have to begin with some type of physical activity. With exercise we will increase the total number of calories that we consume daily, and yet be able to keep on losing weight.

5. Soybean

The tradition of consuming soy dates from the 11th century B.C., meaning about 3,000 years ago, and originated from the eastern part of northern China.

In 1765 soy was brought to the American continent and it has not come off the menu ever since. The consumer groups are widespread in their beliefs that soy should be used as a nutrition replacement for children, when breast milk is not available, for the women in menopause, and especially for people who are vegetarians or those who are vegans. The reason for this is in particular due to their specific ingredients and healthy effects on the human body.

Soy is a good source of proteins from a plant origin. It also contains 8 essential amino acids that the body very much needs. Soymilk has imposed itself as an ideal replacement for cow's milk because it does not contain proteins and fatty acids of animal origin. Instead it contains unsaturated essential fatty acids that reduce cholesterol. Besides that, soy is an excellent source of B vitamins (Niacin and Foliates) and iron. Plant proteins of soy are supporting the function of the heart and circulatory organs. (Anderson et al., 1995)

Thanks to the rapid rise of new technologies, new studies have shown that soy, despite its very useful nutrients, should be consumed in very limited quantities, and some people cannot or should not eat soy at all. Thus, in the last few years and even recent months, scientific works have appeared that have shown that regular consumption of soy in large quantities, as well as feeding infants with soy milk as a substitution for breast milk, can have serious and crucial consequences:

* Allergies and severe gastrointestinal dysfunctions

* Crashing the immune system

* It can cause growth problems in children

* Phytotripsin in soybeans could intensify anti-thyroid agents that may cause cancer of the thyroid gland

* Soy contains trypsin inhibitors that can compromise the function of the pancreas

* Vitamin B12 in soy is not absorbed by digestion. Instead, soy is even increasing the need for vitamin B12, especially among people who are vegetarians or vegans.

* During the processing of soybeans there is a creation of Glufosinat ammonium that is similar in structure to an amino acid called glutamic acid, and this is a powerful neurotoxin.

* Soy contains significant amounts of aluminum, which is harmful to the kidneys and nervous system.

(Gail Elbek, 09.02.2010; Kaaya Daniel, PhD, 2012, Weston A Price Foundation, 4/30/1999)

6. Cause of cardiovascular disease

The doctrine states that elevated cholesterol in the blood is causing cardiovascular disease, i.e. diseases of the heart and blood vessels. This doctrine has never been disputed. Drugs are being prescribed, specifically statins that are reducing Cholesterol levels. If someone would even think of opposing this theory and practice, it would be considered as pure heresy, and even a medical error.

These beliefs are being scientifically denied even as I write this, and have become a myth.

A few years ago, scientists assumed that the real causes of heart disease and vascular inflammatory changes in the vessel walls are scientifically proven and a paradigm shift has been made in the treatment of cardiovascular disease.

Simply stated, when there are no chronic inflammatory processes in the body, there are no inflammatory changes in the vessel walls. In this case cholesterol will glide freely through the veins and not stick to the walls, which would create a clog. Acute inflammation in the body is a natural body defense against all kind of attackers in organism such as bacteria, toxins and viruses. Chronic inflammation of the body on the contrary is very harmful and leads to heart disease, heart attack, stroke, diabetes and obesity. And last but not least, it leads to cells aging and death.

Chronic inflammation, according to the latest research, occurs partially because of recommendations for decades to reduce consumption of fat in the diet.

This has created shifts in food production by offering low-fat foods enriched with hidden sugars and calories. Only recently have they stated that the only recommended fatty acids are omega-3 oils. Any processed food not only contains more sugar which is then bonded to the protein that has been consumed, but leads as well to chronic inflammation of the vessel wall.

Processed food is cooked in soybean oil and corn oil, which are omega-6 oils. This oil is used to process all products of fried potato chips as well as all French fried products. This leads to an imbalance in the ratio of omega-3 oils, because the molecules of omega-6 fats are essential. This means that they are a natural part of every cell membrane, which is responsible for the permeability of the cell walls.

If the omega-6 fat intake is widely consumed through processed products and prepared foods, then the cell walls begin to produce so-called Cytokines that directly cause inflammation. Omega-6 oil is used very often in cooking processed food because they prolong the life of these products on store shelves. In addition, an inappropriate intake of calories causes weight gain and elevated blood sugar levels, and this creates cardiovascular disease, high blood pressure, diabetes, and even as recent studies have proven, Alzheimer's disease.

The process of chronic inflammation proceeds very slowly and can remain unnoticed for quite a long time. The vicious cycle of consuming processed products closes in on you, every day, more and more.

The only way to avoid chronic inflammation is to not consume processed foods, or packaged food from supermarket shelves, but to eat only unprocessed foods, such as natural steamed vegetables, moderate in salt and seasoned with olive oil or very little butter derived from cattle that feed on pastures.

(Dr. Dwight Lundell, one of the top heart surgeons in the US, The Cure for Heart Disease and The Great Cholesterol Lie, 08/19/2012)

And as we always suggest, use your common sense. If you are consuming unprocessed food, try to prepare it yourself, being moderate in salt, and season your meals only with olive oil. You will not have cholesterol problems either. In the end, you will be on the safe side no matter what the result of the newest major discussion between scientists concerning cholesterol can be.

Chapter 3

Bioenergy

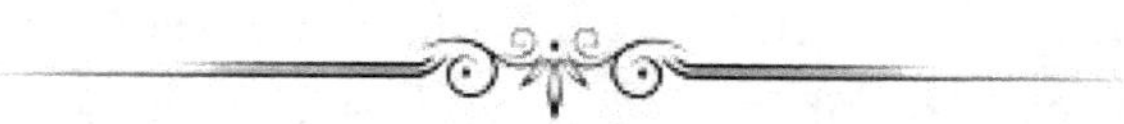

Bioenergy is the life energy, which is, as the name says, part of all living beings. Everything that lives consists of bioenergy, including human beings, animals and plants. If there is no bioenergy, the being is dead.

Bioenergy is a part of the Universe and has been well known for thousands of years. The first written notes about Bioenergy are going back to ancient China, and are described in I Ching, which is translated as "The Book of Changes " dating from 1122 B.C.

I Ching is about the three energies that are crossing each other. These energies are cosmic energy, Earth energy and Human energy. About 300 B.C. many people in China became aware that Human energy could be manipulated in quantity as well as in quality. These people were then helping in the curing of diseases.

It is known that breathing techniques have been developed many, many years ago, but no written notes exist from that time. In about 58 B.C. Buddhism started spreading throughout China. In the very secretive Buddhist monasteries, far away from the masses, Buddhist monks started experimenting and studying very profoundly the techniques of Bioenergy. The techniques that were used and developed by the Buddhist monks of that time were performed on very deep levels trying to influence and control human aging and the Bioenergy of the organs. No written records from this time exist about it, and nobody will ever know exactly how far the monks came in development of their techniques. One thing is sure; they must have been very successful because there are some notes about Buddhist monks from that time living to be far over the age of 100.

Generally, the western world is having a clear stagnation of progress, as well as questionable human integrity, which is having an impact on medicine as well. One of the most disastrous and tragic eras of human history, the dark ages or medieval times, was well known for the inquisition, torturing, suffocating and suppressing of everything that was and might have been progressive, new, having new visions or was liberal. All those who dared at all to think different were simply eliminated.

In the year 1911, the change of the Ching Dynasty took place in China. In the monasteries, many documents and written records that were hidden from the masses

of people, and were coped with religious rituals, were released and many of these records have become public in later decades.
The basic rules of Chinese medicine have been established on bioenergy.

The progress of the technique and improved communications worldwide has brought to the light of day that similar techniques and documentations existed in other parts of the world as well. These areas include Japan, India, and the Middle East to mention only a few.

The development of bioenergy in the western world has happened relatively late in history, which is not so strange considering that the interest in Chinese medicine first started with Acupuncture. This treatment was a breaking point for Chinese medicine and many people in the western world became interested in it. Acupuncture became very prevalent in the 1970's.

Despite the fact that the healing methods of Acupuncture and Bioenergy Healing are very different methods, they have in common the same kind of energy that is all around us.
The numbers of Healers have been increasing all over the world ever since. There are people that exist who have a special feeling for diseases without being psychic. They have healed other people around them

by applying Bioenergy, without even knowing it exists.

As the western world progresses in science and medicine, they will acknowledge only what is visible and can be proven. So Bioenergy did not exist for them because something that you cannot measure and make visible on instruments simply does not exist.

Albert Einstein was also famous for his sayings, many of which will gain relevance as time passes. In his office the following quote was pinned on the wall:
„Not everything that counts can be counted, and not everything that can be counted counts. "

Chapter 4

Electromagnetic Waves

"The day science begins to study non-physical phenomena, it will make more progress in one decade than in all the previous centuries of its existence."

Nikola Tesla (1856 - 1943) Physicist, chemist and mathematician

Electromagnetic waves are all around us.

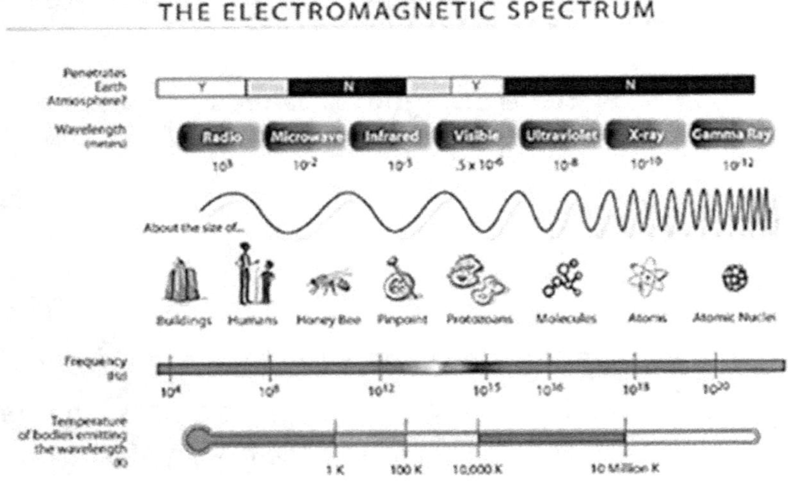

In the mid-19th century, William Gilbert discovered the polarity of the magnet, and many researchers began to perform experiments with new discoveries such as electricity. In 1856 Mr. Maxwell provided a theoretical description of electromagnetic (EM) waves. To produce these waves and to prove them in the experiment, the frequency of the EM waves produced by the oscillator must have been equal to the frequency of the speed of light. However, such equipment did not exist.

20 years later, Heinrich Hertz succeeded to show a connection between EM waves and light, and proved that the waves can be created and spread through space.

However, globally, the first documented EM waves were

the contribution of **NikolaTesla** in his laboratory in Colorado Springs, USA in 1899.

As part of these experiments, Tesla found that the resonant frequency of the EM waves is equal to 8 Hz (Hertz), precisely 7.68 Hz, proving that the resonant frequency of the Earth is also 8 Hz.

In the year 1950, scientists have proven the existence of a cavity around the globe, which extends a distance of 80 km from the earth's surface to the atmosphere and reaches the ionosphere. It is called the Schuman Resonance Cavity.

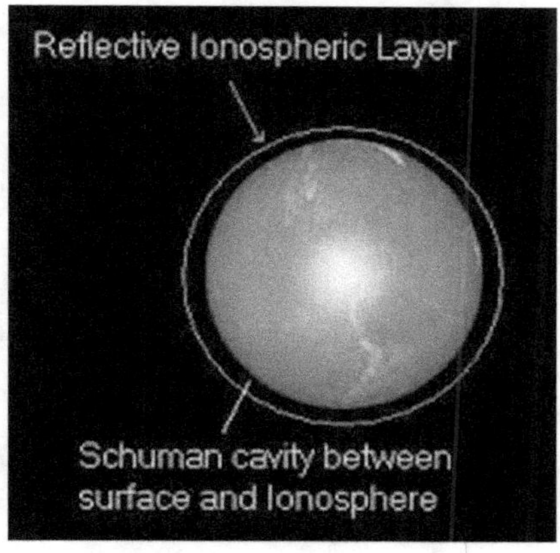

The Schuman cavity is not constant in the speed and spread of EM waves. The factors affecting the cavity at different speeds and intensities of the EM waves are different electrical conductions of the Ionosphere, the difference between night and day, the difference in the magnetic field of Earth as well as absorption of the waves at the poles of the earth, etc.

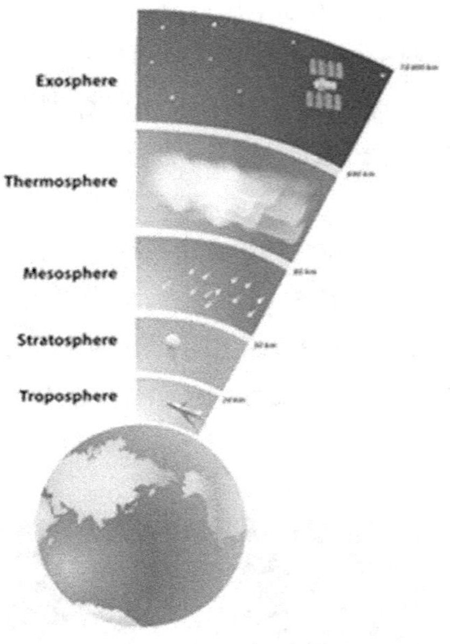

Brain waves

Neurons of the human brain flicker or oscillate at different frequencies or waves without ceasing. Each of the dominant frequencies occurs in various particular situations.

Alpha brain waves were first detected apart from other brainwaves after a scientist, Dr. Berger, invented the electroencephalograph (EEG). These waves were named after the Greek letter "alpha", which is the first letter of the Greek alphabet and have exactly the same frequency as the Earth and the cavity around it - 8 Hz. Sometimes they are called Berger's wave in honor of the inventor. These are the most significant waves because they are found when someone is in a relaxed state of mind, for example in meditation.

It is a state of mind where a person is fully awake, but very relaxed and is aware what is happening around him locally. In this state, the mind coordinates the work of both cerebral hemispheres, removes stress and depression, and stimulates imagination and creativity.

Alpha waves have an optimal frequency when people, who are awake, have their eyes closed. Alpha brain waves do not exist until the age of 3 years, and recent scientific documents show Alpha waves are used in different forms of communication.

(Palva & Palva, Trends Neurosci, 2007)

Alpha brain waves are our subconscious, where all our programs are stored in the brain as a complete operational capability of one individual.

So how do we bring ourselves into a state of Alpha waves?

There are people who can manage their brainwaves in certain situations and are considered gifted. But other people, who do not have such innate abilities, can develop this skill by targeted exercises. One of the methods that is recommended and which will be discussed later is a method of visualization.

Ideal conditions for Bioenergy Therapy are when both the therapist and patient reach an Alpha brain wave state.

Man has the power to create using the power of thoughts and thinking. "What the mind of man can conceive and believe, it can achieve" is one of Hill's hallmark expressions.

Hill, Napoleon (1937). *Think and Grow Rich*. Chicago, Illinois: Combined Registry Company. p. 14. ISBN 1-60506-930-2.

Here are other brain waves and their frequencies.

* Delta waves (0.1 to 4 Hz) - a state of deep sleep / dreams
* Theta waves (4 to 7 Hz) - the dream state, the area of hypnosis
* Beta waves (12 to 30 Hz) - normal waking consciousness
* Gamma Waves (25 to 100 Hz) - transcendental meditation

The brain continually produces waves at different frequencies and by doing so determines the state of the mind.

Delta waves are very slow and low in frequency, and are the deepest stage of sleep (REM).

Theta waves that are slightly higher frequencies appear in the dream state and represent a state of deep relaxation and peace. In this state it is possible to implement hypnosis. Some psychologists are calling Theta waves the boundary between the conscious and the subconscious, which holds memories, feelings, experiences, and the beliefs that define a particular person.

There is an immediate transition from Theta phase into the Alpha phase, which begins at a frequency of 7.65

Hz. In the range of frequencies between 4 and 11 Hz, meaning the Theta and Alpha phase, behavioral patterns can be changed.

Beliefs are deeply imprinted here at the border of the conscious and unconscious, so that the creation of new affirmations and desires can be effectively and successfully undertaken. But this only occurs when the brain comes to the frequency of Theta and Alpha waves.

Beta waves are the normal state of consciousness of a person who is fully awake. This state is where he is analyzing, assessing situations and is highly affected by mental tensions. Looking at someone in their daily rhythm, the healthiest time is the transition from Delta to Theta waves. During this time, one is in a state of slow awakening - Alpha waves, and only then, the transition to the Beta waves should occur.

Practical Applications

In everyday life, it means that one should not jump right out of bed, like being on springs right after awakening. The best thing you can do, as you become conscious of being awake, is to stay a few more moments in bed, opening and closing your eyes several times. After that you should stretch properly to shape your Aura around your body.

After coming to a fully awake state, then you can get up using normal movements.

If you use an alarm clock to wake yourself, then the preferable alarm system is an alarm clock with a radio. If you prefer a normal alarm clock, be sure to choose one that has a low volume buzzing at the beginning of the function that is increasing with time.

Always use the snooze feature. Modern alarm clocks have a snooze button; so set the alarm a couple of minutes prior to the time you need to be fully awake. That way you can stay in bed till the next signal triggers and get up when your brain waves have transitioned from the Alpha phase into the Beta phase smoothly. You will see that by improving your awakening experience, and graduating your brain frequencies slowly, you will have a better start in your day and everything will be easier.

Gamma waves are waves or vibrations with frequencies between 25 and 100 Hz. Gamma waves are the frequencies of the brain that are named after the Greek letter "Gamma". I want to mention that there should be no mistake that they have nothing in common with the concept of Gamma Radiation! While emitting gamma waves, our state of mind is considered to be perfect. The mind is totally calm and relaxed, but alert.

Gamma frequency wave experiments have been conducted on Tibetan Buddhist monks in a state of deep meditation, specifically transcendental meditation. It has been shown that, while in this state of mind, the brain releases endorphins, and that, because of this release, these frequencies are having a restorative impact on the body and bringing clarity to the mind. Most of the tested Buddhist monks have had gamma wave frequencies between 30 and 42 Hz, which is the highest measured frequency of modern day.

"The entrance to the Transcendental Meditation is hard work," said the Dalai Lama, who is spending 4 hours every morning in this kind of meditation. "I am waiting for scientists to find a faster and easier way to get into it."

O `Nuallain Journal: Cognitive Sciences, 30.05.2009
M. Kaufmann: Meditation gives brain a change: Study Finds, 03.05.2010

Bioenergy and Scalar Waves

Bioenergy has been known by many people for thousands of years and has been transferred to the various cultures and regions of the world under different names.

Chi, Ki, Prana, Pneuma, Brahma, Akasha, Orgon, Bioplasma, Mana, Mungo, Baraka, Bioenergy, Scalar Energy are just some of the names for the same type of intelligent energy.

Bioenergy is scalar electromagnetism.

Scalar waves are electromagnetic (EM) waves, which are a new physical entity that surpasses all comprehension of frameworks in classical physics.

Nikola Tesla, one of the greatest minds and innovators, had an extraordinary insight and intuition. Between 1899 and 1900, in his laboratory in Colorado Springs USA, he made an immense contribution to the progress of the classical theory of dynamic electromagnetic field.

Those contributions have been precisely formulated by British physicist Clerk Maxwell (1831 - 1879) in the form of partial differential equations,

Tesla has managed to produce experimentally a scalar

wave through his powerful emission device, which is named after the part of Maxwell's equations that were written in scalar form.

A scalar wave is defined in basic terms as a complex electromagnetic - gravity (EMG) wave with strange properties. By that I don't want to say that these are supernatural properties, but rather, complex natural phenomena of general scalar waves in which the EM component of G is equal to zero. It has been scientifically derived from Einstein's General Theory of Relativity concerning super relativity in four-dimensional 4D hyper-space-time discontinuity.

Simply stated, scalar waves can be distinguished from electromagnetic (EM) waves and gravitational (G) waves in that they are expanding into the hyperspace or 4D space. It is composed, in contradiction to our material 3D space and the world we live in, from 4 independent spatial dimensions – the three dimensions plus time. Therefore one of the main characteristics of scalar waves is that they can move through space and through time.

There are no material barriers that can stop the scalar waves. The only exception is the special geometric shaped bodies, made of dielectric material that are attracting each other under certain conditions while refracting and focusing. These areas of science are a matter of research for many scientists. These unusual properties of scalar waves significantly complicate their detection and measurement.

But in certain circumstances scalar waves, unlike gravity (G) waves can be misused in different ways. This is exactly the point where scalar Electronics have entered the area of top secret and strictly confidential military physics.

In his research Nikola Tesla has discovered that scalar waves are moving through 4D space and are only occasionally touching the reality of our three-dimensional 3D world. He also found that the maximum speed of the scalar waves is the speed of light.

But because movement of waves in 4D hyperspace is not limited in time, the waves are spreading almost instantaneously. Spots or cracks where 4D hyperspace briefly touches and enters into our 3D space are the door into a 4D hyperspace.

That touch is actually the exchange of energy flow and is taking place via virtual photons that have a zero mass and are unstable. So when those virtual photons skip into our 3D world in which we live, they are due to its instability and quickly returned into the higher energy state. This movement creates actually *a scalar wave* or *torsional field,* which is the Russian term for the scalar wave. When two or more such places, where the 4D hyperspace made a "door" or a "hole" in our 3D space, so called "tunnels or worm holes" are created. Through these tunnels someone can send signals, energy, or can even travel without loss of time (interstellar travels).

Using Bioenergy Therapy as a treatment in which the body can heal itself is happening exactly as the principles of energy waves discussed above. This is also the place and way how distance bioenergy therapy is able to occur.

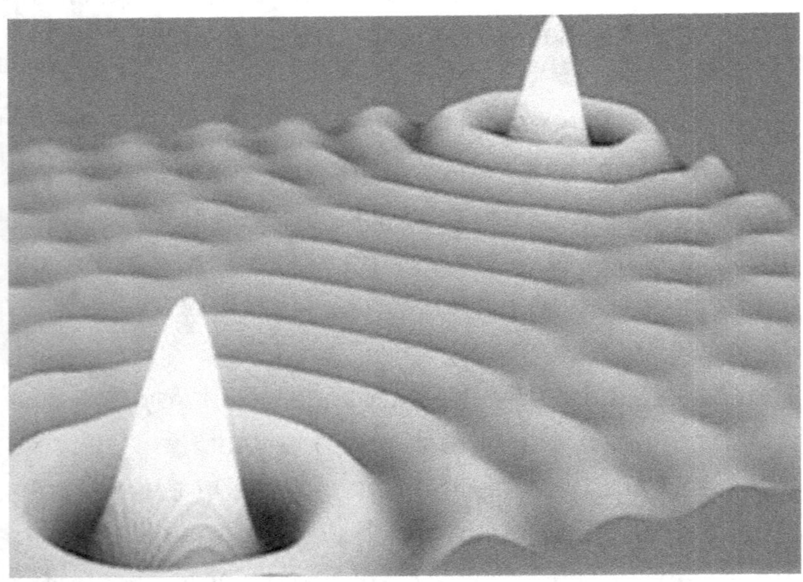

Chapter 5

The Application of Scalar Waves

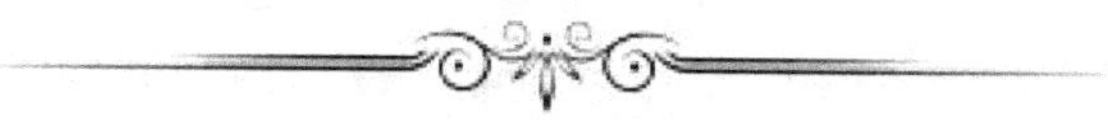

Lightning balls of Nikola Tesla

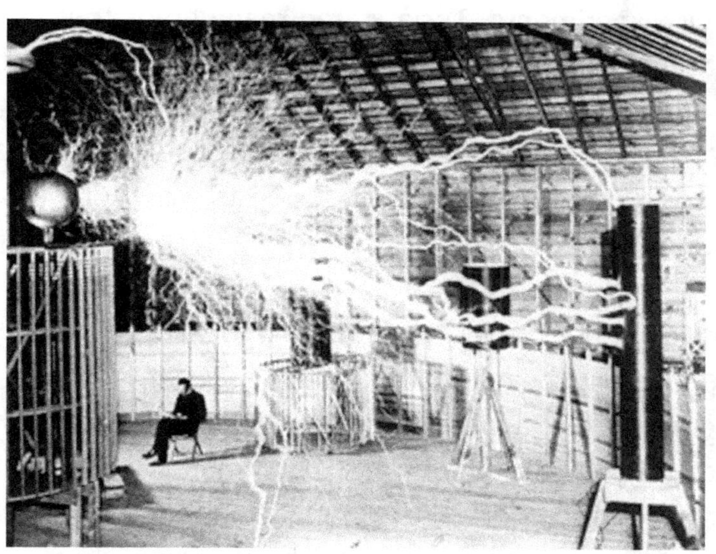

After the death of Nikola Tesla in 1943 in New York City, many of his research records, notices and drafts, that are still the subject of research, came to be missing.

Tesla had always talked about the inexhaustible source of cosmic energy and possibilities of their use for peaceful purposes, as proven by his experiments on a powerful broadcaster in his laboratory in Colorado Springs. In this experiment he used high-voltage high-frequency resonant transformers, better known as the "Tesla transformer", to produce scalar waves. These scalar waves were responsible for the appearance of lightning balls, still scientifically unexplained.

In his speeches that were held during the presentation of his experiments, Tesla stated many times that he did not want his discoveries and free energy theory to end up in abuse. But his discoveries have opened a new chapter for the weapon industry to develop a weapon that exceeds everything that exists now or will be developed in the near future.

The audience in his presentation would listen to his speeches with admiration and disbelief, not nearly understanding what he said and what Tesla had become aware of during his experiments. He said that his experiments are the turning point for all mankind. He was aware of the fact that his experiments were very far ahead of his time, and once said: "The present is theirs, the future, for which I really worked, is mine."

Based on Tesla's sketches, which remained after his death, scalar energy was applied for the first time in an experiment named "Philadelphia" after Tesla died in 1943 during World War II. Other experiments in scalar wave technology that were later performed were called

"Montauk" and the HAARP project.

Having lived during the time Tesla made his experiments, Albert Einstein had knowledge of the many Tesla experiments, and the development and modifications of those inventions. Albert Einstein confirmed many of Tesla`s experiments, saying on one occasion: "I do not know what weapons will lead the third world war, but I know what kind of weapon will be used in the fourth world war - sticks and stones."

Philadelphia Experiment

In 1943, when the war intensified and was at its height on all fronts, the U.S. Navy performed experiments with the military ship USS Eldrige. The goal was that the ship could become invisible to radar, using knowledge about scalar energy. Producing scalar waves based upon the plans of Nikola Tesla, the ship not only became invisible to radar, but also was remarkably beamed into the port of Norfolk for a short time, 320 km away.

The shock and disbelief become greater when the generator that produced the scalar waves was turned off. The hand of one of the sailors was embedded in the steel hull of the ship, basically "poured" into the steel.

The effect of scalar waves erased the borders of the real and unreal. Many movies were made concerning this experiment, and the happenings described, after the Second World War. These movies were made into a story format, but, in reality, the basic theme exists, in that Tesla's experiments were embellished.

But this shock continues when we become aware that Tibetan yogi Milarepa performed something very similar in the 11th century BC. He was able to produce scalar waves during which he imprinted his palm directly into a stone.

Project HAARP

I want to describe Project HAARP only briefly as a contribution to a better understanding of the application and operation of scalar waves, i.e. cosmic bioenergy.

This project is called the High Frequency Active Auroral Research Program - (HAARP).

With the application of scalar waves in the framework

of this program, which was one of the first of its kind in the development of scalar waves, it has led to changes in parameters such as chemical structure, temperature and humidity in the upper atmosphere. Specifically affected was the atmosphere at a height of 50 to 80 km, which contains a large amount of charged particles, upon which its name was given, Ionosphere.

The project has actually initiated the era of the manipulation of the climate on Earth.

Today's development of electronics, technology and the technical possibilities has dramatically exploded in the last 20 years. It is possible to produce rainfall, storms, tornadoes and even earthquakes.

So why are all those scientific, liberal and politically relevant groups on this planet wondering why global warming is occurring?

One of the reasons for global warming is certainly air pollution. There are numerous, mighty and expensive symposia, reports, lectures and conferences about how the main cause of climate changes are human's carelessness and pollution of the environment.

Without any doubt, this is true. But is it whole truth? No, it is not, not by far.

The HAARP Program is the U.S. government's most controversial project ever undertaken in the whole history of America.
The project incorporates proven scientific experiments on the creation of a protective shield around the Earth, and these experiments penetrate below the surface of the earth into depths that have never been seen before. It also can be used to develop incredible weapons of mass destruction.

Who is behind the project HAARP?

With the exception of the experts in the fields of physics and mathematics, the U.S. Air Force, the U.S. Navy, the University of Alaska, and the Defense Advanced Research Projects Agency (DARPA) jointly fund the project. The DARPA is responsible for the development of new technologies for use by the military. For ordinary people these are very mysterious forces in action.

In reality, these are powerful people in governments, who consider themselves the elite, and thus owners of everything around them, including our existence.

Why was the HAARP project really made?
It was obviously made so that the respective groups and lobbies of certain forces could use it for military purposes, but has become a very scary method to

control many other factors of our lives. Google "HAARP", or visit http://www.youtube.com/watch?v=iRN0GDFH3Vs to find out more information.

Successful films of science fiction, such as "Star Trek", have been produced in which utopian scenes appear that might happen at some point in the distant future. But for now, it is just information, artfully displayed science fiction, and nothing more. When we get out of the movie theater, the illusion ceases and we return to reality, in which unfortunately, there is not much room for the truth. The truth is that we in fact could set ourselves free from their control.

Technology and weapons that already exist today and are being produced in secrecy are portrayed to the general public as just another illustrated fantasy for the wide masses in films such as Star Trek. This way the truth is belittled, made unrealistic and laughable.

And the truth looks as follows: In the best case, the HAARP is a high-sophisticated science, which got out of control. At worst, it is an unknown weapons technology or futuristic technologies that incorporate it all, from the weapons on the super-Rays to the equipment for the mass mind control of the entire world.

Positive use of bioenergy

You cannot always measure all that is important and not always all that important is measurable.

Albert Einstein

If the technology of scalar waves, or cosmic bioenergy, is used for peaceful purposes, it goes far beyond the imagination of a human being and possibility of anything that has been seen before. It brings freedom, free energy, antigravity force, and thereby is reducing the pollution of our planet Earth. Most importantly, Bioenergy is applied in the treatments and healing of all diseases, including all forms of cancer.

Simplified, but so far the only known healing explanation, is that scalar waves are forcing the damaged cells to return to a healthy state and therefore the time of illness has been reverted to an earlier period.

Otto Warburg, a Nobel Laureate, said: "The cancer cell has an amperage of 15 mill volts, the old cells have amperage of 50 mill volts, and normal healthy cells have amperage of 100 mill volts. Every cell in the body has a small battery inside. When the battery runs out, which happens mostly because of stress, damage or disease, you have within yourself a problem with electricity."

Life energy or Bioenergy has been always present in the universe and has been known for a relatively long time. It is a kind of intelligent energy, which, if properly applied, leads to healing by filling up the cells that are out of energy. Bioenergy exists in all living beings, humans, animals and plants, and works on all levels: molecular, cellular, organ and the whole organism.

The God's Code

Scientists working on *bioenergy,* which is essentially a *scalar electro-magnetic theory,* developed something called the "string theory". This theory assumes that everything in the universe, from galaxies to subatomic particles, is made up of tiny lines of energy in the form of strings. These strings form the String Theory.

The String Theory is not only a theory of everything; it is also a theory of time and time travel. The newest developments in theoretical physics suppose that time travel is possible trough the wormholes. The whole Universe is vibrating and so are we as well, thus everything in the Universe is a matter of frequencies.

As of now, the energy that would be needed to pass

through a "wormhole" would be a Planck-energy of 10 billion electron Volts.

The latest math of "creating energy" has proven that the world, as we know it, is not complete. Besides the 4 known dimensions (three-dimensional - 3D space and time), it is believed there are 11 specific dimensions. Nobody yet knows what kind of shape those dimensions form. These discoveries have contributed to science and common knowledge in that we know that space is far more dynamic and changeable then even A. Einstein thought. The Universe can be stronger then anybody could have imagined.

The biggest minds of our time are working on String Theory. One of them is Edward Witten from the Institute of Advanced Study, who made a significant contribution to a String Theory lately. In his studies, he was able to merge 5 equations into a single common String Theory and called it M-Theory (which stands for magic, mystery or matrix). M-Theory is bringing our Universe on a very thin membrane, or as they call it in the world of science "the brane". It is assumed that there are many such membranes, which are parallel to each other, i.e. there are many Universes parallel to our Universe, but we cannot see them or enter into them because the brane is not permeable. This Theory brings us to also look at the problem of gravity on a very different way.

It is a breath taking vision.
If the String Theory is regarded from the aspects of a mathematician or a nuclear physicist, those dimensions can take on any kind of tens of thousands of forms, and each of these forms fits into its own universe, having, accordingly, its own physical laws. In the world of Science, it is always a problem how to prove the claim.

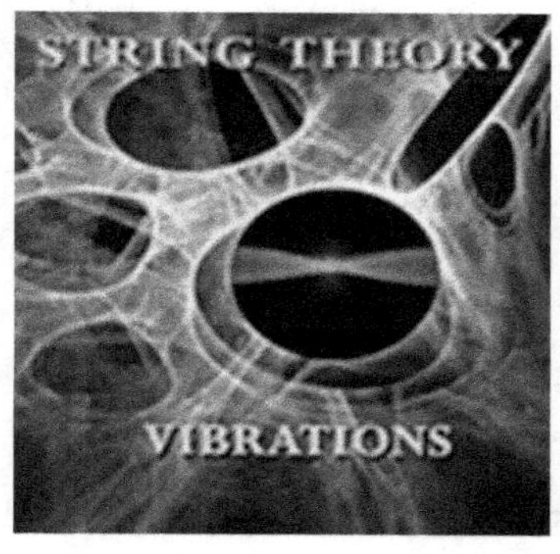

If the "String Theory" could be proven, or rather, when it is proven, it will reach the *critical point of string theory,* and it will be evidence of a *"theory of why everything exists,"* or, as they call it by another name - **the God's Code.**

The Field of Positive Intentions

Bioenergy, i.e. scalar waves, are responding to our *intentions.*

A vast quantum energy field of scalar waves connects the universe. Thought generates its own palpable energy, which you can use to improve your life and these thoughts become your intentions.

If we move into a space where there is a void and not even a dimension of time exists, we create a scalar field. This scalar field is overcoming everything. It will lead to the collapse of the field of reality in which we exist in our three-dimensional world. When that field of reality collapses, it leads us to the second field of reality that is aligned with your intention. And exactly here, the limits do not exist anymore. By that I mean all the boundaries, not just time, do not exist, and anything is possible. Healing through bioenergy becomes reality. We will discuss tools in how to achieve this scalar field as a state of mind later.

There are of course elements that influence the success of treatment, such as quantity of the bioenergy fields (scalar fields) that the healer has. That means that the healer acts as a conductor, and is able to accomplish an internal constraint, or the ability to realize his intention for the treatment of Biotherapy and accomplish the work successfully.

Tesla was also convinced that scalar waves, i.e. Bioenergy, are having an influence on thoughts, and conversely, that our mind is able to create scalar waves, i.e. Bioenergy. These waves reveal to us the true dimension of the universe in which the human being is only a small but inseparable part. Our experimentally proven perception of the reality in which we live is that we exist in a three-dimensional material world, and this is just one part of the Universe, which is connected over higher dimensions, both materially and spiritually.

This is also the basic premise on which bioenergy fields are based, and that exists around every living being and is called **Bioenergy.**

Development and Recent History of Bioenergy Treatment

On the opposite side, quite the opposite of evil, a good prevails.

Bioenergy is around us, within us, and all around us. You only need to apply it.

That was also the working theory of a project by Trieste born scientist *Antoine Priore,* who was an electrician and a radar technician in the French army. Based on thousands of experiments, which Priore performed in the 60's and 70's of the last century, he used an electromagnetic device for animals. He has proven, with nearly 100% effectiveness, that he can treat infectious diseases, diseases of the immune system, leukemia, all cancers, as well as other diseases. The results of these treatment experiments were published in 1960. When a shift in the French government occurred in1974, Priore has lost most of the proponents that had supported his work in the previous government, and also lost his financial backing. Thus most of his works were "lost."

The French government, as stated later by scientist *Tom Bearden,* "finally came to the realization how a scalar electromagnetic wave can be applied to create weapons more powerful than any nuclear weapon can be."

In addition to *Tom Bearden,* who designed and patented the "Motionless Electromagnetic Generator" (MEG), a Russian by the name of Lahkovsky had fantastic success in cancer treatment and healing of broken bones with bioenergy. *Lahkovsky* worked most of his life in France. His very simple devices were used in hospitals before the Second World War, but suddenly they were "missing" because of "unknown causes."

One of the pioneers in the treatment with bioenergy that continue to develop *Tesla's* initial discovery was *Dr. Wilhelm Reich.* He is of Austrian origins, escaped the Nazi regime and fled to the USA. He worked there on the development of bioenergy, which he named "Orgone".

He also developed devices for the modification of climate and developed a machine he called the "cloud

busters", sluggers of the clouds. He called this research "Cosmic Orgone Engineering", and it was successfully implemented in a drought in Maine during 1953.
He was just one of the few who have tried to apply bioenergy, as a source of free energy in the service of man and our planet. He was arrested by the U.S. government, and his works have been destroyed, books burned, and he died in prison, reportedly of a heart attack.

Today, 70 years later, there have been blowing some other winds and a new era has arisen. The methods of Biotherapy treatments are still showing disbelief, but there is, on the other hand as well, a kind of tension among those who are engaged in offering of treatment - the bioenergy therapists themselves.

One thing is definite: it cannot be denied that Bioenergy Therapy has a healing effect on our bodies.

A certain group of people appeared who continued researching, studying, developing and application of Bioenergy Healing Techniques, where their predecessors had left off 70 years earlier.

Their path was full of doubts, rejections, ridicule and accusations. They had to fight hard and stand up for themselves and their beliefs for a long time, in order to get where they are today. All this just because they managed to prove that the methods of bioenergy are healing diseases which have not yet been shown to be possible in scientific experiments. And maybe this is what makes them what they are today: in good and bad.

Today there are many Biotherapists worldwide. Some of them are calling it "Quantum Healing", not only because it has roots in Quantum physics, which is a study of physical forces, but also because it is connecting the Biotherapy Methods with science, giving it an allure of significance.
But whatever the name some of them are giving to Bioenergy therapy, or the effort to make a brand out of it with their own names included in the title, there are many therapists worldwide who are successfully performing their treatments and contributing to the energy movement that is going to set mankind free.

Nowadays, Bioenergy therapy has spread over many countries and continents including the US, Ireland, Russia, Turkey, Switzerland etc., to name just few of them.

In the not so distant 70's of the last century, these were individuals who had confirmed their success on hundreds of thousands of people, some of whom owe them their lives. But in the constant struggle to survive and defend their methods, these creators of the clinical application of Biotherapy, have personified themselves in the roles of Guru and demigods. Nowadays, when they are standing there at the end of their life's work, they are leaving behind, not only a valuable legacy of their treatment methods, but also the human imprint on which they should not be proud of at all, and which has certainly removed them from their carefully constructed throne. But it's hard to live by the principles that we are preaching to others.

How to Choose a bioenergy therapist

As with any other type of therapy that you are intending to use, the rules to visit any medical office are always the same. Between those who are giving the treatment, i.e. therapy, and the one who receives the therapy, i.e. the patient or client, there must be implemented a kind of communication, as well as human and social compatibility. It's called rapport.

Rapport includes not only the sympathy and admiration; it also has a mental link between the therapist and the client. There is an expressed or unexpressed seed of confidence, which is so important that it is an absolute requirement for you to decide for therapy by this particular person and place. Recommendations are obtained, and confidence is gained. One of the criteria is that you must feel comfortable and be ready and willing to give confidence to your therapist so that you are going to be a source of information for your therapist that he will need in order to provide you with a successful therapy. This is the main precondition for the creation of rapport, i.e. for good and successful mutual cooperation. Over time you will gain some experience and you get a feeling for how to choose a therapist, no matter what the treatment is about. If you have not succeeded in doing so, do not criticize yourself. The one who is successful is the one who always gets back up on his feet after falling. Keep on going.

Healing with Bioenergy

Bioenergy is an energy field that all living beings, humans, animals and plants, possess. If Bioenergy does not exist, then the person, animal, or plant is dead.

The definition of being healthy in medical terms is the absence of disease. By definition in holistic medicine, *optimum health* is a balance of mind, body and spirit. *Bioenergetic medicine* represents a state of optimal health. This is expressed in the smooth flow of bioenergy to achieve balance in the body. Thus harmony and coordination between body, mind and spirit is achieved.

We are speaking here about the concept of *optimal state of health*, because a perfectly healthy person does not exist, nor is there a man who can live forever or always maintain the "ideal" healthy stage. Balance or equilibrium permits the free flow of bioenergy, which not only has to be done effortlessly, but must be in constant motion.

Bioenergy will freely flow throughout the whole body. However, when the paths of bioenergy are blocked so that the energy flow is interrupted or even stopped, there is an imbalance of bioenergy in the whole body, which then leads to disease as a result. The disease begins to develop long before the start of the noticeable symptoms.

Bioenergy existence has been proven, but it is not measurable. Bioenergy effects are visible for now only on the *Kirlian photography* and *Gas Discharge Visualisator (GDV).*

More about Kirlian photography can be found at http://www.kirlian.com/.

Bioenergy leaves an imprint on the DNA, boosting the chemical components within the DNA and thus makes it more resistant to damage.

Bioenergy also has a clear impact on our thoughts, which are, as well as all other energy vibrations, an untraceable and invisible field of the Scalar Zero Point.

Chapter 6

Bioenergy Medicine

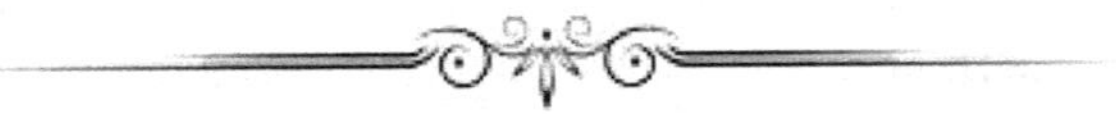

Levels of the human being

There are three levels of a human being that make up the whole. These three levels must be altered in order to obtain a complete harmony where Bioenergy flows freely. This way the body will take control for the protection or treatment of itself, depending upon its needs. In this way the body, as a whole, keeps itself healthy by the coordination of all three levels.

1. Physical health - This can be effectively influenced by the way we choose our diet, physical activity, getting sufficient sleep and regular care and attention to our body. This level means that we have proper physical hygiene for our body and care for it is as a kind of shell since it is the only one we have.

2. Mental health - Consciousness is a psychological emotional condition in which we have optimal control of our minds awareness. Proper mental hygiene means we are actively controlling our thoughts. If our thoughts are irrational, they are not under control. The main goal

in the maintenance of our mental health is to get rid of "mental trash".

3. Spiritual Health - This can be influenced when the subconscious is released and is then having a positive impact on our consciousness. This is the information that is reprogramming the subconscious. The very first step in this direction is to clear any doubts you might have.

Only under the condition that these three levels are in balance or harmony, can we speak about the healthy condition of the human being.

Physical health and diseased conditions

We can always do something for ourselves in order to feel better. We do not necessarily need to be sick to be concerned about our physical health.

Physical health has to be coordinated with the other two levels of a human being, mental, and spiritual health.

Disease or a diseased condition first appears at the level of the psyche and within ones thoughts. As soon as a human being is in a state of stress, fear or anger, the result is the secretion of adrenaline. This will cause a chain reaction that will result almost immediately to prevent the secretion of certain hormones and chemicals in the body that are responsible for the positive influences on the mind and body, such as Serotonin, Interferon, or L -dopa.

The message is clear. We cannot afford to have negative thoughts. When we are thinking about our particular problems, we are creating scenarios that might possibly never happen and are really just a pure illusion. If we allow these situations and illusions to overcome us and to last for a longer time, this can create such devastation in our body that will certainly far exceed our original problem. The price is simply too high for negative thinking.

According to the latest research, our body communicates within itself through chemical components such as *Neuropeptides* (NP) and *Cytokines*.

Until recently it was thought that only the brain produces NP, but it was discovered and proven that all cells in the body communicate through Neuropeptides and act as the acid in the battery that powers the starter. Then chemical reactions in the cells are converted into electrical energy. This all happens in microseconds. The human body and cells exchange information between each other and transmit positive and negative impulses through NP and Cytokines. Then our mind starts to cooperate with the endocrine system. In this manner, the immune system is put into action and has been mobilized.

Does that sound like Sci-Fi - science fiction?

An event occurred at the beginning of September 2012, while I am still writing this book. A Post Office in Zürich Switzerland, which has a huge facility located on the edge of the city and has hundreds of employees, was caught by surprise when a package with white powder and a threatening letter was found. It was not clear whether the chemical was a poison, a bomb or something else. The news spread rapidly through the huge complex. When some of the staff began to develop signs of suffocation, severe coughing, vomiting, allergy on hands, fainting, etc., which required immediate medical intervention, crisis management was created. Finally they decided to evacuate the entire building. The employees, visibly upset, started to collect on a parking lot of the facility, and medical management teams were assisting to keep the people warm, although it was not too cold of a day in late summer, with tea and drinks.

Thirty employees were urgently transported to the hospital. The results of the analysis of the suspicious powders have shown that the white powder was only

edible food starch. Just the suspicion and fear that they were poisoned was sufficient to make a significant and medically relevant change in their medical condition in a large number of people.
Here you go - rumors and the negative thoughts by the employees became a reality show.

Therefore, our goal should be to develop a method to block the input for the stress of any kind before the neural transmitters cause a chemical reaction that is detrimental to our bodies. This stress could be generated from fear, anger, doubt, thinking about difficult situations, feelings of guilt, or destructive messages.

A disease as a result of the negative impact of stress, fear, or anger is then searching for the parts of the body, organ or system that have the lowest electrical potential of the cell. Chemicals, such as *Serotonin* or *Cytokines*, reduce even more the electrical potential of the cell, and this is exactly the place where disease occurs. Of course, there are certain types of diseases that are having their outbreak because of genetic heritability.

Scientists who are trying to find a cure for a particular disease or group of diseases are then creating a syndrome and that becomes a name for the disease. Medications that have been found and developed for certain diseases are curing the symptoms only to a certain degree, meaning they have a limited effect and duration. This treatment by medicines did not affect the cause of the diseases, which were created as a result of stress at the level of the mind. The disease is then coming back again with its typical symptoms. Once consumption of the drugs has begun they cannot be terminated without consequences (e.g. medication for high blood pressure, antidepressants, anti-high Cholesterol etc.) Therefore, the disease cannot be eliminated by any kind of pill or removal of that part of the body.

The exceptions are quite something different. Medicine and doctors are successful in all emergency situations, such as appendectomy, acute abdominal surgery in accidents of all types, breaking of bones, emergency room situations, and so on. Therefore medical treatment in all types of emergencies is acceptable and self-sufficient. In cases of disease, however, this is not yet true.

Desperate people in their despair often turn in prayer to God. They pray alone or in groups in the presence of more people in a church. Prayers, like certain music or mantra, are repeating certain mystical sounds, such as a mantra that is repeating the essentially recognizable sound, AUM. This creates a particular resonant frequency and if it lasts long enough that the body and mind are merged into one resonant rhythm, a Field of Positive Mental Intention (FPMI) has been created. I have named it here the Field of Positive Intentions, and should not be confused with the technique of positive thinking. When a person creates a Field of Positive Mental Intention, it must have a purpose, commitment, eagerness and devotion. When the intentions and commitment are bigger, it is easier and quicker is to achieve the FPMI.

The Field of Positive Mental Intention is essential for healing of any kind. Therefore most of the people who are being treated must mentally accept this treatment. Otherwise the cell activity is inhibited. Inactive cellular activity blocks the production of neurochemical compounds that are inducing the immune system to work and allow the free flow of Bioenergy.

This is the basis for further development of Neuroimmunology, and hopefully in the near future, the development of Holistic Neuroimmunology. The latest research in the field of Psychoneuroimmunology has proven beyond a doubt that expressions of kindness, love and positive support activate healing energy at the cellular level. Disease results from interaction between the cells of the human body and the mind, and the "pattern" or code that is created in the mind of the person cannot be removed by medication.

This means that the body and mind of human beings together represent an unusually sensitive bio-electromagnetic machine.

Energy Medicine acknowledges the energy that a subtle life force or a life triggers. The strength of this energy determines the state of human health and well being. All living creatures radiate a frequency of the energy that is generated by oscillations. All organs have their own energy frequency.

The goal is to maintain healthy cells in the equilibrium of the natural vibration frequency and ban the frequencies made from the emanation of energy from cells that are coming from germs, bacteria and harmful pathogens, which are having their own energy vibrations. In this way reprogramming of the vibrations of the unhealthy cells is taking place.

Everything that lives has its own optimal dose of vibration. This optimal dose is called resonance. When we are in resonance, we are in balance.

AURA

Aura is the emanation of energy surrounding the body of every living being in the universe, including man. It is displayed as a subtle radiation field around the body, which is spreading like a cloud to a distance of about 70 cm around the body.

For people who have special senses, which we call then a synesthetic person, the Aura is visible in a spectrum of colors that surround the body. Auras have different colors and different meanings. A damaged Aura indicates that someone could have some disease.
Aura is also called a biological field, or a "Human Energy Field."

Aura consists of electromagnetic particles, microwaves, infrared waves and ultraviolet light. Depending on the spectrum, the waves have a certain frequency. Lower frequencies, such as microwaves and infrared waves, in which body heat is expressed, are associated with the bodily functions of DNA, circulation and metabolism. The higher-frequency waves, such as ultraviolet waves, are associated with conscious activity such as thinking and emotions.

The perception of Aura should not be connected to the perception of the human Astral body. An Astral body consists of electrons, more precisely 4 billion trillion electrons, 4.0 times 10 to the power of 21. Each electron has a memory, and it contains information. The astral body transmits and receives messages by means of these electrons through the brain without us being aware of it. It exchanges information with our higher self during sleep. The saying "The night brings counsel" emerged from the common experience that some people often have the solution to their problems upon waking in the morning. Hence the term "sleeping on it" came to be.

For more information please visit,
www.nujournal.net/choice.html

Aura is different in color and shape depending on the situation and on the characteristics of the individual.

The form of the Aura has a different thickness and is enveloping the body like a silk cocoon around caterpillars before they are hatched as butterflies. Some are calling it an "Auric Egg." If the aura is interrupted, there is a deficiency or imbalance of bioenergy on that part of the body, and if it is too thick, it can mark the location of a problem area with an excess of energy. Excess energy is often a cause of pain and has to be removed by bioenergy therapy. Some interpretations are based upon the premise that an Aura has 7 layers corresponding to the number of Chakras on the human body. Upon this theory, each Chakra is corresponding to one layer of the Aura, and respectively is connected with each other at the Chakra point.

Interpreting the meaning of the colors of Auras is a very important instrument of diagnostics. A Synesthetic person who is trained in the interpretation of Auras can see the physical state and mental health of the person under observation.

The color of an Aura can vary in the parts around the body by the color and the intensity of the color. The emanations can be very shiny or dull as a mist, and can also look like reflections in the Aura. If the reflections during the observation of Aura are quickly changing in color, it means that the person's thoughts are changing rapidly.

The general meanings of the colors of the Aura are listed below:

Blue - Indicates a relaxed person whose nervous system and psyche are balanced. These people are prone to survive at all costs. They are ready to help the others around them, sometimes spending too much energy in the process.

Green - Describes a person who has the gift to be a healer. This person has a "Green Thumb" so that everything grows in their garden.

Yellow - Indicates a person of joy, who displays a sense of freedom or Independence. When it is part of the aura around the head, yellow indicates that the person is or can be a spiritual leader. It is believed that Jesus and the Buddha had such a color in their Aura around their head.

Orange – This is a sign of mental strength with the desire and the need to control others. If the orange color is blending to yellow around a person's head it indicates a person who is a powerful spiritual leader.

Red – This is a person who has a very strong commitment to the material world and their thoughts are focused on the physical body. A person with red Aura knows what he wants and can be stubborn.

Pink - This color is rare and occurs in the form of flashes in parts of the Aura, and is connected with the person's thoughts. These people are having harmony or balance between the spiritual and the material matters.

Brown - Indicates that a person is unable to decide and materialistic oriented.

Ochre/mustard – Indicates a person who suffers from pain in his physical body and they are full with rage.

White – A sign that a person has a severe illness or is using some kind of drug. The physical body and the mind of the person are not in compliance and not in balance. White color Auras appear a few hours before the person will die. In many cultures with ancient traditions, Death is shown in white, and the people who are mourning for the dead person are wearing white and not black clothing.

The only two methods that can prove and show the Aura are the Kirlian method and the Gas Discharge Visualization (GDV) invented in 1996 by Prof. Korotkov from the Technical University in St. Petersburg, Russia. In recent years, the program has been computerized in order to provide a quick diagnosis. The computer screen will show the Auras of the person's fingers. Different areas of the fingers are corresponding to different organs in the physical body and mind of the person. Using this technology, the health status of individuals can be determined.

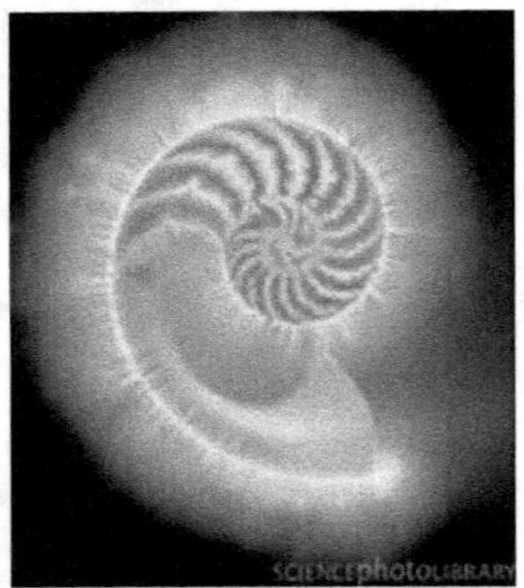

For those who want to learn more about it, visit www.kirlian.com

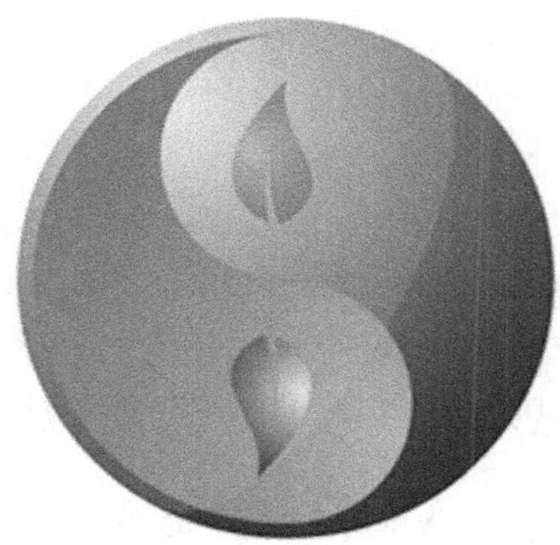

Yin and Yang

Yin and Yang is the principle of Taoist polarity that exists through the power of different polarity in harmony. It is based on the I Ching, translated to English as "Book of Changes", and is the oldest Chinese cosmology and philosophy recorded dating back between 2,000 and 3,000 years B.C.

Yin and Yang are based on differences that are opposing each other, in close relation to each other, thus in perpetual balance and proportion of equal forces, but their polarity leads to mutual attraction and creates an energy pair. They are not permanent and are always changing, and are in an eternal relative state attracting each other. Only in this way the principle of the universe can be realized.

Everything in nature is based on the law of Yin and Yang. In nature, a child's conception, Yin (egg) and

Yang (the seed), are meeting together.
The flower stalk is solid and straight (Yang), and the flower is soft and round (Yin).
The cup is solid (Yang), and the tea is liquid (Yin).
A house is Yang (solid structure), and the atmosphere in the house is Yin (feelings).
A cup containing water is half full (Yang) or half empty (Yin).
The human body is Yang from the outside and Yin from the inside of the body. And every human body has its own separate Yin and Yang.
Bioenergy or Qi is Yang, blood and bodily fluids are Yin.
For the ant a man is huge (Yang), for the universe a man is tiny (Yin).

Yin and Yang must be in balance in order to keep a body in a healthy condition. If they are not in balance, then disease occurs.

When death occurs, Yin and Yang are going apart.

The body and mind can endure a relatively long hectic and stressful day (Yang), but when you are not careful and are not paying attention to interrupt stress with periodic breaks and relaxation (Yin), then a diseased state will occur

Nothing should be done too little or too much. The rule of moderation in all things is the golden middle.

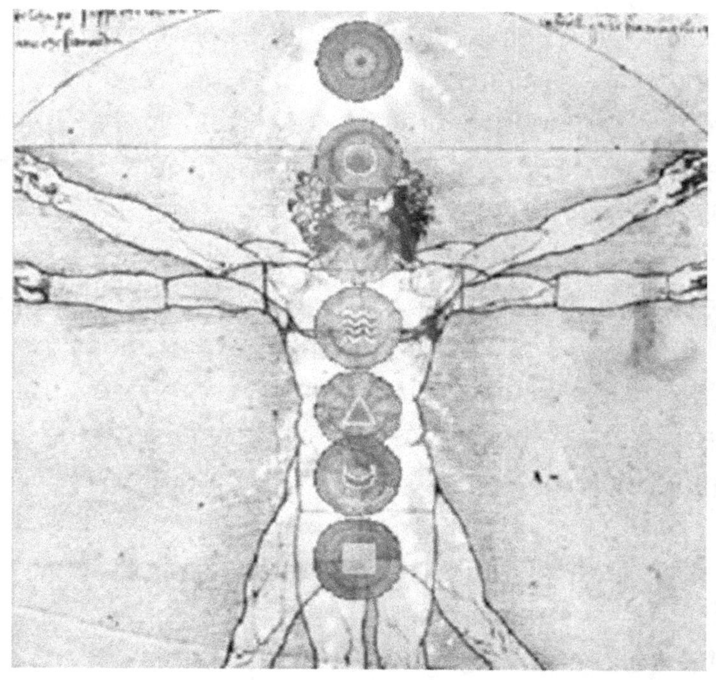

Chakras

Chakras (pronounced: cha:kras) are the centers on certain parts of the body where a person collects energy. The name Chakra comes from the Sanskrit word that means a "wheel" or "roller". Chakra, as a concept, is appearing in many techniques and philosophies, especially in traditional Yoga and in the traditions of Hinduism and Buddhism. Chakras were introduced to the Western culture and the Western world relatively late, first in the early 20th century through translations of Indian texts and records.

Through the strong similarities between the two philosophies, Chinese and Indian, Chakras are incorporated in the practice of Acupuncture, as one example of a Chinese Medicine that uses this philosophy.

The teachers of the modern era and the movement called "New Age" have, by their explanations of the Chakras, used computers as a comparison. Major Chakras are compared as a hard drive. Each hard drive contains a lot of files.

Chakras are described as energy centers that are placed in a straight line on the body, going from the pubic bone and ending with the last or seventh Chakra on top of the head. Chakras are thus associated with certain organs and glands. The New Age movement also associates a certain color with each Chakra.

The function of the Chakras is to turn and twist the Bioenergy clockwise giving to each center a free flow of Bioenergy (Chi, Ki). In this way, the mental, emotional and physical health of a person's body is balanced. In the case of a malfunction, energy is flowing in the opposite direction, or counter-clockwise. The intensity of the disease is in direct relation to the intensity of the disturbance or wrong flow of energy by each certain chakra. This explains why people that are having chronic diseases that last for longer periods of time need longer bioenergy therapy treatments. In that case, the disease has left the psychological imprint.

A great importance is given to the Chakras in the psychic relation of the person, but also the physical relations are taking an important place as well.

The names and the location of the Chakras:

1st- Root Chakra - at the end of the spinal column behind the pubic bone

2nd- Sacral Chakra - in the middle of the lower abdomen

3rd - Solar Plexus Chakra – either behind the navel or the solar plexus

4th - Heart Chakra - on the chest above the heart

5th - Throat Chakra - the lower part of the neck in the area of thyroid

6th - Third Eye Chakra - between the eyebrows

7th - Crown Chakra - the top of the head

Immune System

The immune system is a system of biological structures in the human body that protects the body from disease. When fully functional and without error, the immune system prevents a large number of different pathogenic agents to have a negative effect on the body. The immune system can prevent diseases ranging from bacteria and viruses to parasites and fungi, while at the same time distinguishing diseased tissue from healthy tissue. The science that deals with the study and investigation of the structure and function of the immune system is called Immunology.

About 70% of the biological structure of the immune system is located in the gut. The other 30% consists of white blood cells or leukocytes. This is also understood to be the general or non-specific immune system.

There are three barriers of the non-specific immune system, i.e. mechanical, chemical and biological.

The mechanical barriers include the skin, mucous membranes, coughing and sneezing, and rinsing activities of body fluids such as tears and urine.

Included in the chemical defense barriers are antibacterial enzymes that are contained in saliva, tears, and breast milk.

The biological barriers are considered to be a flora in the digestive tract that has the ability to, if necessary, change the environmental conditions by changing the pH. This allows reduction of the number of pathogens that could be developed in the numbers required to cause the disease.

If one of the pathogenic agents is able to cross all three barriers, then it spreads around the body by developing various reactions to the poisons. The immune system is reacting and responding to the attack, in that it remembers and recognizes the pathogen if it appears again in the body, and creates antigens or antibodies. This is called immunological memory, or an acquired immunity.

One of the first responses of the immune system to an infection is inflammation. This means that the immune system defends itself by causing an inflammation, and the body will develop all five symptoms of inflammation: fever, redness, pain, swelling and loss of function.

Signs of inflammation are the result of actions by Cytokines and other chemical substances that the immune system is releasing as a response to the inflammation, sending immune cells to the site of the inflammation to allow healing of the damaged tissue. Inflammation, therefore, is not in itself a bad thing.

It becomes dangerous when the inflammation is repeated so many times that the immune system leads to a condition that it not only weakens itself, but may also lead to the point where it can "break" the system from functioning. It then starts sending cells that are attacking its own body, not recognizing it as their own, but is considering it as a pathogenic agent. As an example, there are a group of diseases that are very dangerous, and largely incurable by medicine, called autoimmune diseases. This condition is where the immune system attacks its own body or its organs.
As of now autoimmune diseases are not treatable through school medicine. All autoimmune diseases are successfully treated and completely disappear or show a significant reduction in symptoms and relief by Bioenergy Therapy.

Two other groups of diseases of the immune system are enfeeblement or inactive immune system (e.g. caused by AIDS or certain cancers), and hypersensitivity of the immune system.

An inactive immune is as dangerous as an overactive immune system. When the body is weakened through lack of sleep, eating excessive junk foods, and other damaging factors, the immune system is weakened. This can be a life-threatening situation. So it is important to lead a balanced life through proper physical health.

Hypersensitivity is divided into 4 types depending on the severity of allergic reactions.

The first group has a very pronounced allergic reaction that can be life threatening and must be treated urgently and immediately. An emergency room is the only place where they can and must solve such cases.

The second and third groups show less dramatic reactions to the stimulus of the immune system and the reaction can take 2-3 days to develop.

The fourth group is a very weak reaction, or no reaction at all, that can create an imperceptible inflammation. An inflammation can eventually become a real danger to the body and be attacked by the immune system, and can therefore create an autoimmune disease. One such example is the constant inflammation that occurs in the digestive tract, and is, for the most part, caused by food intake on which there is hypersensitivity. This means that there is an inflammation existing, but it is so weak that the cause could not be immediately determined. Such constant inflammation in the gastrointestinal tract, caused by a hypersensitivity to a particular food, can lead to serious disease and consequences, especially if the person is having a diverticula in the colon, and not aware of this condition.

You need to know that about 60% of the world population is afflicted with intestinal diverticula. But when these mini-inflammations persist without treatment, and under certain genetic preconditions, it can lead to very serious autoimmune diseases such as Crohn's disease and celiac disease.

A test called Cytolisa - Test, or ELISA procedure, can be performed in every major laboratory by specific blood tests to determine intolerance to a particular type of food. The obtained results show a list of about 200 types of food, which have a concentration of antibodies to a specific food, and are shown in the graphic colors. It is helpful, because it clearly indicates what food must be avoided and not be consumed at all.

Hypersensitivity to certain foods can be healed with 100% success by Bioenergy therapy.

In any case, it is highly recommended to take Enzymes because that way you are supporting the body's ability to digest the food. More about enzymes, their activity and usage can be read in the chapter about nutrition.

It should also be noted that one of the main factors for the proper functioning of the immune system is ultimately Vitamin D. It has been proven that the aging of the body leads to a lack of vitamin D, which is in a symbiotic relationship with the function of the immune system. Do not let a single day pass without taking vitamin D.

Self-control of the mind and how to achieve the Field of Positive Intention

The mind is the creator of everything. Your mind controls every action you take and any situation in which you are.
Your own thoughts must be kept under control. This can be practiced with some effort. From the moment we wake up, our thoughts swarm in our head. Some of these thoughts possess us and we cannot get rid of them. Then we let the thoughts continue swirling inside of our heads throughout the day in the hope that they will stop obsessing us and we will eventually get rid of them. However, we need the conscious part of the mind for everyday life.

Imagine your mind is an airplane. It has a pilot and copilot. The pilot represents your conscious mind, and the copilot represents your sub conscious. When the plane is flying on autopilot, your conscious mind is not working, and you are not controlling the information that is coming into your brain. The conscious mind is busy somewhere else. That way, the paths to our subconscious, are wide open to all kinds of information around us because our awareness barriers that should be controlled are not working any more. It is in this state, our subconscious mind is open to all the information that is pouring into it.

When our mind is in a heightened wakeful state, it is operating at 134 bits / second. Our conscious mind is registering about 8 bits / second. Our subconscious mind works at a speed of 210 million bits / sec. The subconscious mind works continuously, registering all events around us without the ability to influence the information we receive. A classic example of this is aggressive advertising - billboards that are placed every two hundred meters along the highways. Do you believe that you have not noticed a single detail? You are wrong - it is registered in your subconscious.

Or, for example, we start thinking about a particular problem that preoccupies our daily existence, wishing to reach a solution of the problem that way. But the thoughts we create are in relation to the basic problem of the situation, which is not real because it has not yet occurred or happened. We then begin to interpret our thoughts without using rational thinking on which the basis of good decisions can be brought. This occurs because the thoughts cannot see into the future since they take place in a space that contains a dimension of the past, so that the thoughts have been transmitted or are projecting the past into the future, assuming that history must repeat itself. And the truth is that the only thing we have is the here and now.

There are techniques, one of which is *self-hypnosis,* to *stop* your negative *thoughts.*
How many times have you started to say something, and then you say, "Oh, I forgot what I wanted to say "? In a similar way, some thoughts may be interrupted on purpose. You start visualizing an item, which has been pre-selected, for example an apple. So if you find yourself with thought that are driving you crazy and cannot get rid of, just make the conscious effort to think of this apple, so that your thoughts are channeled in a different direction.

Only in this way with daily exercise at a randomly selected time, visualizing about this specific item and using it as a trigger or *turning point* in the cessation of thought, you will be able to bring your own thoughts under control.

Later on, you will be able to turn back to your problem and then rationally decide to make a decision about how to finish something, how to do something, or how to react in a certain situation, etc.

Thoughts are irrational, if not controlled.

Only those people, who manage and succeed to break through the barriers of the negative programming of their mind and create a field of positive intention, can be "pulled out" i.e. saved.

The Field of Positive Intention does not consist only of positive thoughts. As a matter of fact, it has nothing in common with the term "positive thinking". But it consists rather from being able to bring your thoughts under control. Moreover, you need the commitment and fascination for the subject of your intentions and a strong belief system. With a strong Field of Positive Intention, and a strong belief system, you can heal anything.

The Field of Positive Intention operates optimally in measurable EEG frequencies. These are the frequencies of brain waves, vibrating in a range between 8 and 30 Hertz, namely Alpha and Gamma brainwaves. The last are achieved through a transcendental meditation, and during their vibrations or oscillations, cognitive achievements at high levels are possible. An example for this state of mind is when we are so focused on something that we lose track of our surroundings, and the people around us are getting the impression that we are in a daze.

Tibetan monks, who have collaborated on studies of transcendental meditation, have described their state of consciousness as extreme wakefulness, although from the outside it seems like they are completely submerged in thought. When measuring the brain activity of Tibetan priests, psychiatrist Dr. D.R. Davidson, has discovered that besides the fact that all of them had brain frequencies above 30 Hertz, the neurons in the brains had been synchronized like clockwork.

Meditations and Contemplative Neuroscience

The Tibetan monks, that were part of a project on researching transcendental meditation, have described their state of mind as very conscious and alert, despite that outside viewers were having the impression that they are immersed in their thoughts.

Psychiatrist D. R. Davison, M.D. at The University of Wisconsin in a joint venture with Dalai Lama, performed the measurements of brain activities of Tibetan monks. Two Groups were part of the experiment. The first group was made out of 10 students that had no experience in meditation. The second test group consisted of 8 Buddhist monks that had spent the majority of their lives, between 15 and 40 years, in meditation.

The two groups of test subjects have shown very significant differences on instruments that measured their brain waves. The Buddhist monks have shown high frequencies of Gamma brain waves – between 30 and 42 Hz. The test group of students reached barely the lower margin of the Gamma brain wave frequencies, i.e. 25 Hz.

The results of very high Gamma brain waves that had never been measured before at that level, stayed constant by the Buddhist monks for a longer period of time after meditation, i.e. their Brain waves lasted longer in difference to those brain waves measured by the test group of students, The results of this test have shown that a meditation performed by Buddhist monks has led to a neuroplastical change on their brain structure.

Except of the fact that all of the Monks have developed Gamma brain waves higher than 30 Hz, it has been discovered that the neurons in the brain had synchronized impulses of functioning. This further promotes the integration of the brain neurons.

MRI Imaging Techniques have proven the existence of the brain structure changes. The brain cortex is getting thicker, in that it is increasing its surface but getting more curled as well. This is called *girification*. It is happening because of the increased number of synapses as well as capillaries that are playing an active role in supplying the brain with oxygen and glucoses.

Meditation that is practiced by the Buddhist monks, as well as Dalai Lama, is called transcendental meditation (TM).

Upon explanation of Dalai Lama, it is a state in which the care and maintenance of mental hygiene is being taken care of. According to Dalai Lama this is not state of mind, but a state of being.

This means that if we are training the state of consciousness of our mind we would be able to maintain and perform the hygiene of our mind. The purpose and the goal are to delete and reject all mental trash.

The mind can be trained very effectively with this kind of mediation as **Yoga In Connection with meditation**. In this kind of meditation, Alpha brain wave frequencies have been measured that have been very stable under outside disturbances or interventions.

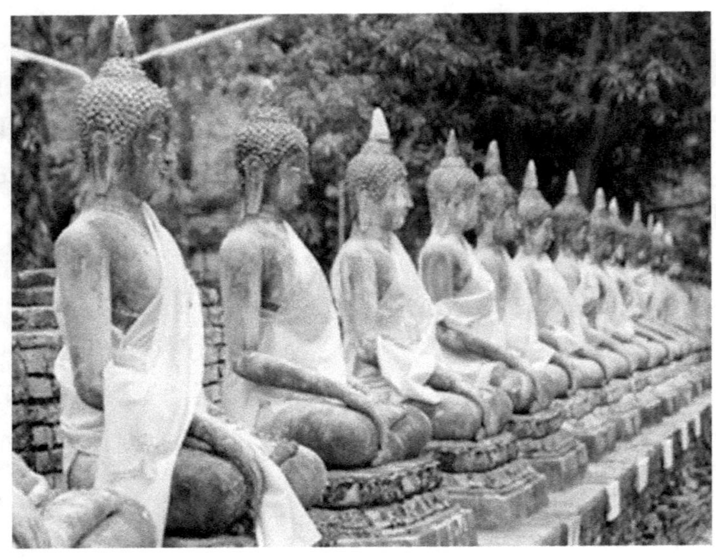

Zen meditation is a Japanese form of meditation, which is expressing itself in the brain waves frequencies of Alpha brain waves, measured by an EEG. The neuroplasticity of the brain is with this kind of meditation achieved with an encumbrance (kurou). The encumbrance is the fronting of a new idea in a form of a puzzle, which is resulting in an increase in the number of neurons in the brain. At the same time, Zen meditation includes pain, because it is said, that there is no neuroplastic improvement without pain.

Contemplation is a mental kind of practice in which thoughts are separated from everyday life, and occupied with something different or devoted to something else, which we admire, for example God.

Almost all religions are having contemplation incorporated in their religious practices.

How to Change yourself

It is said that if you believe in what you are doing, it will come true. Not always. If you have not assorted the things on your "hard disc" - i.e. carrier of information in your subconscious, then only believing in what you want to achieve and are doing is not enough.

People can change, but the only way to do this is to change themselves. You cannot change the environment or another person, but only yourself. However, this way you become a different person entering a new life, in spiritual terms, which is as a result opening the way to balance. This is to give you a reason to do this, and you will be surprised to see the impact it will have on your environment, motivating other people you are connected with to change themselves. A good example for this would be that a person, as a part of his education, training or company support would visit a psychologist. Even after the first session, his partner at home would notice the changes being made. The partner would ask, "What happened to you? You are so different today". It has to be understood that a psychotherapist did not change the person; they inducted the subconscious of the person,

and motivated them to change. With some small but very useful techniques, you can also do it yourself. You will reach transformation for the better, which is your final goal in your life.
Man's thoughts, like all other energy vibrations, are at immeasurable fields *of a scalar zero point.*
Modifying and controlling your thoughts are having an impact on DNA, in that the chemical bonds within DNA become resistant to disease. This is opening the paths and flows of bioenergy within the body.

Working on oneself is a difficult and demanding job, which primarily requires great discipline. The vast majority of people prefer to leave their consciousness and everyday life on autopilot, which means that they allow their conscious to be driven by their subconscious. As they would say in America, many people just "Go with the flow". The first step towards the liberation of the information of the subconscious mind, which is damaged or reprogrammed, is to understand the illusion and erase any doubts.

The worst enemy of any transformation is the refusal of reality and living in an illusion. Many people live under the illusion of happiness and love, and they do not really know what love is. Some people suppress their emotions, because they do not know otherwise, and are just being fake. Love is learned from parents or guardians and is learnable until the age of 4. People who are not lucky enough to grow up in a properly functioning family have really no idea what love is, and are considering love as a feeling of gratefulness or as a feeling of being needed. If they become brutally shaken in their illusions, then they are convinced that there was no love in the first place. But they simply cannot know because it is not possible to identify something, which is not recognizable.

We have invited all players to enter into our lives. But that does not mean that they have to create pain, illness and emotional chaos.

Very often it is said that some people "think and are guided by the heart." Or better known - "My heart tells me that...". This is a completely wrong belief.
These are people who actually have no control over their emotions.

If you're the type of person who does not tolerate conflicts so well and would rather run like hell or you cannot deal with certain problems and conflict situations and jump on the first ball, then stop, wait, and sleep on it. The most effective thing to do is to go for a walk close to where you live in the park or around the lake. You should take at least 30 minutes to an hour, or about 3 miles. During this walk, you should sort out the thoughts that were occupying you, and not make any decisions, other than thinking about when is the right time to carryout the solution, which will be effective. This is not easy and we need, first of all, great discipline, self-control, confidence and determination.

This is what marks the decisive and successful opponents.

Consequently, and especially if in your situation it would be reasonable to ask an expert for advice, or simply someone smarter than yourself, which has nothing to do with the level of education, it will open up new possibilities for actions and solutions. However, if you act or react immediately to the situation, then there are only two possible responses. These are to either "fight" or "flight", better known as "Fight or Flight Syndrome". This basically means to actively defend yourself, or to flee as far as possible i.e. "Get the Hell Outa Dodge".

Referring to the above, there are two types of people: those who have an outward orientation and are thinking they always have to be accepted by others, and those others who are introverted. They do not care what others think about them and if they receive any negative feedback from their environment, it will not affect them and will not faze them unless the feedback is equal to or greater than a Tsunami.

Besides that, generally you have to be aware that something that you are persuaded of becomes a part of your reality. And, in your subconscious, it creates programs that govern your life. Perhaps you control the people around you unconsciously believing that the world as you have created is all right. "I'm fine just the way I am". This is an illusion that only you alone can solve.

If you are not satisfied with your life as it is now, at any level - whether it is your health, your mood, interaction with other people, the immediate environment, your partner, children, parents or partner at work, interacting with other people in the immediate or wider environment, your business success which is very important, because it is the basis of proving yourself, but it is also a very important source of your income that feeds you and your family - then you live with the illusion that everything is alright with your life as it is now. You cannot see it, because it is safer to stay in this state as it is now, than to do any changes and thus engage yourself in something unfamiliar. You would prefer to stay in pain than to change anything, because of the fear that, with change, the conditions would be worse. Change is always a flight into the unknown.

One of the goals is to exercise in letting go. You must allow yourself to accept other opinions and concepts without judging them, whether good or bad. But to start with, you should be very cautious about incoming

information, i.e. disinformation messages that you receive every day. Later on or with time, you are going to be able to be deferential to them in a split second. This is just a matter of exercising.
Hidden information is nevertheless sneaking into our subconscious at a speed that we previously found to be unbelievable but true as we mentioned earlier. So we must be on the alert to protect ourselves from manipulative information. The way to protect us is to learn to visualize. This means that we imagine in our thoughts we have a kind of a shield and we are watching it as a movie scene. The best thing to do is to exercise at the beginning of every day for a couple of minutes. An example of a shield could be a shield made out of steel, which is protecting us from the other side, or a glass dome under which we put ourselves. I personally prefer a glass dome because I can watch what is going on outside the dome, and at the same time I can invite inside whomever I want to offer protection. This is a good example of a tool in protection of children, older people, or pets. With our closed eyes, we are watching ourselves inside a glass dome running a scene in front of our "third eye". In reality, it is a chakra placed on the forehead between the eyebrows. In our thoughts, we are repeating "Reject, Delete, This is none of my business".

We are never involving ourselves in any kind of inner discussion i.e. some kind of inner conversation between yourself and the incoming information, because this would consequently lead to a defense reaction and activation of adrenaline. After that you have as described before, only the two possibilities, Fight or Flight. So you have to select very cautiously everything you think, say or do. And also at the same time, be very selective and cautious toward things that others are telling you. Anything of that can be programmed into our minds. We can handle it only if we know how to neutralize it or to delete the negative inputs or information.

This is the way to slowly but surely increase your self-worth, self-confidence and your self-value. That way the people around you are starting to experience you differently.

The newest scientific works in the field of cellular microbiology and quantum physics, which are still a matter of intense research, are showing that the cell walls or membranes contain a specific protein called IMP, Integral Membrane Proteins. They are reacting on the indirect exchange of bioenergy inside and outside of the environment. This result in scientific research has a huge value because it is proving that the biological changes of the cells can be influenced with invisible sources of energy, including thoughts.

If we are able to block our inner thoughts, we are

concentrating ourselves on meditation or prayer. In this manner, we are opening ourselves toward this subtle energy which is everywhere around us. Because this energy, which is Bioenergy, is also affecting our DNA, it is affecting all levels of our body and mind that are running all our body and mind processes. This is how we are able to heal ourselves.

We are all connected with a source of bioenergy, which is at the same time, creating the universe as well.

We all need resources that would enable us to fill up with energy when we need it to find inner peace and relaxation. While looking for resources for meditation towards a path of a self-reconnection of self and knowledge are Runes and I Ching.

Both ancient arts come from very different people on the planets. Runes originate from Scandinavia, and I Ching is coming from China. It is possible to spend very pleasant and entertaining moments, and at the same time, undertake a serious rehabilitation on yourself.

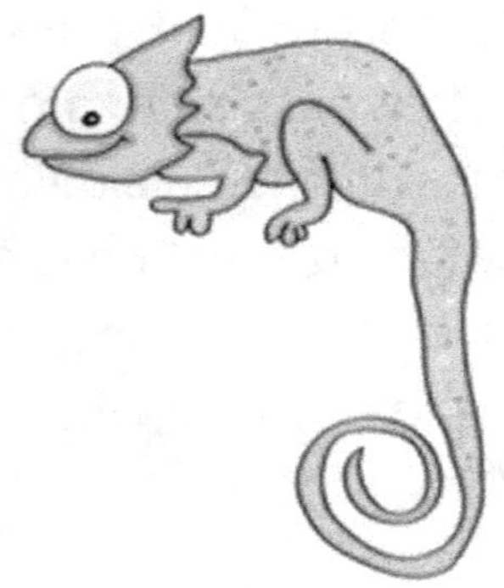

Take a look for more information on Runes and I Ching at at http://bioenergy-balance.com

If you are not in a position to go for a walk and help yourself on that very simple, but very effective way of "first aid", you can help yourself in many situations of your mind and body that is requiring attention with a technique named *Jin Shin Jyutsu.*

If you are, in despite of everything, having a feeling that you need help from outside please consider treatment by a high profile hypnosis therapist.
http://hypnosetherapie-schweiz.com

Chapter 7

Bioenergy Therapies

What is Bioenergy Therapy?

There are many kinds and forms of Bioenergy Therapies. Some of them are effective in that they are helping the body to heal itself, and some are useful as a support for the body, so it can reach a state of equilibrium or balance. This creates an improved balance physically and mentally for that person, which gives this person a good feeling of being healthy.

To begin learning Bioenergy Therapy, you should first examine and test your own abilities in order to determine whether you can create an optimal state of mind. This is a prerequisite and is a must for any kind of bioenergy therapy to be effective. Having the proper mindset is in itself the beginning of the bioenergy process in the human body, both as a therapist and as a patient. That way you are enabling your body to be accessible for bioenergy.

If you find that your state of consciousness cannot be realized, and needs more than you can accomplish on your own, or you simply need to re-examine your abilities to see where you are at, I recommend that you visit a specialist for Medical Therapeutic Hypnosis.

Being a practicing bioenergy therapist, many of my patients have realized that their physical disturbance or disease is gone through the treatment. Many of them have battled with their health problems for years, and now they are feeling better. They have reported that they are in a better mood, realizing the difference from before and after the treatment. Yet, they started the process of differentiating and fine-tuning between their body and mind, and many of them have come to the conclusion that they would also try to improve their mental health through medical hypnosis treatment.

Everywhere in the world, this valuable method of hypnosis therapy has been defamed by mass hypnosis exhibitions in large halls where an enormous number of people are inducted into a state of trace en masse. So, what now? What good does this type of show perform? What is the purpose of such a blatant misuse of hypnosis? In the first place, it has absolutely nothing to do with medical hypnosis therapy. Medical Hypnosis is something infinitely more than just the term "to hypnotize" someone. In Medical Hypnosis Therapy we are not "hypnotizing", we are inducing the person into the trance.

Look for an experienced expert in Medical Hypnosis in

your town or area.

If you find yourself in a situation of a medical need which you are encountering daily, and for which you don't need to call an ambulance or go to the hospital, then the technique of **Jin Shin Jyutsu**[R] can be used to help yourself in a number of health conditions. In case you decide for this treatment to treat a chronic or serious illness, be sure to visit a licensed therapist for the Jin Shin Jyutsu method.

Bioenergy, as I stated before, is a kind of intelligent energy, which enables the body to heal itself. Those that are performing the therapy are conductors of energy, because they are directing the energy that is available all around us towards the person that they are treating.

The number of bioenergy therapists, as well as the number of methods and techniques is huge. As in any profession, there are, unfortunately, some people who call themselves healers and have brought the many valuable techniques and methods of complementary and holistic medicine into the realm of doubt and disbelief by their superficial treatments. There are those, of course, who only use their so-called treatments for quick profits and charlatanism, and are nothing more than a fraud.

Therefore, you should carefully choose your Bioenergy Therapist. This book should also assist you with that. Your approach to cure yourself must be obvious and clear, before and during a therapy. Try to repeat before every treatment twenty times: "I *can* heal myself." That which can be believed, can be achieved.

First, be aware that you are opening yourself up to something that's already inside of you, your own life energy. Nobody is giving you no more or no less than the pure energy that is around all of us in space. Everything is already within you. What you need to do is to open your mind, and come to the realization that your body is able to heal itself.

How many times have you heard or found yourself saying: "I believe in - something," or conversely, "I do not believe in it?" The fact is that we ourselves are the creators and producers of our own health. Your intention is to achieve a *state of chronic health*. And with that intention you are ready to go to a healer or therapist. It has nothing to do with any belief system, and especially not with faith as a religion. You are aware of the fact that it is possible to achieve a state of chronic health and are choosing a therapist who will help you to do so. To achieve this you do not need any special place: the largest and the brightest Temple is within the person himself.

In everything you do, even with the intent to create a state of chronic health, it is important to remain reasonable and not create any illusions.

Bioenergy therapy cures all diseases. Yet, in your healing expectations, you should remain reasonable and realistic. Bioenergy treatment for a damaged spinal cord will not be cured, but it will make that person feel better and to cope better with her or his life. This person will find the best way to compensate for this new situation and make the best that she or he can out of the situation. Bioenergy Therapy can especially help those persons who are partially seized by their upper extremities and they can significantly improve the use of their arms. This has a tremendous value for a disabled person. It makes them more independent and self-sufficient in many everyday situations. And even the most minor improvement for a disabled person that can assist her or him in their life can be very major to them. Just think of the Paralympic Games.

Many patients decide to begin bioenergy therapy only when they have already tried everything else, or when school medicine "gave up on them". They were told that there is no further medical help for them and that curing is not possible any more. They come to the bioenergy therapy in very poor psychological condition. They feel "scrapped" and this is, you should agree, not a very favorable condition of consciousness. As a matter of fact, it is very different and opposed to that state of mind in which a person should be in, as I described in previous chapters. For a cancer patient, their physical condition is of course far from optimal: the organism as a whole, the organs, cells and components were either destroyed or significantly weakened by progression of growth of the tumor cells, usually after one or more Chemotherapies.

It is important to make a decision to begin the bioenergy therapy as early as possible.

Personally, I decided for myself to take bioenergy therapy for a viral infection. The bioenergy therapy that I received lasted more than 6 months and did not have any success. Today I know that the intention of the therapist, or the laying of his hands on the affected part of the body, is not enough for a patient to achieve a free flow of vital energy, or bioenergy. Not to speak of the situation when a patient is in pain, which means that the area of the body has accumulated too much additional energy in the painful area, and the healer is adding even more energy on top of that. So it is no wonder that it is not working.

In today's era of the awakening of the human consciousness, bioenergy therapists are becoming more and more prevalent, as well as the explosion of communication options. Many Bioenergy Therapists have stated that, no matter whatever technique of Bioenergy therapy is performed or how it is performed, all bioenergy therapies are equally effective. This is not accurate.

How is Bioenergy Therapy Performed?

I have decided to provide a comprehensive description of the biotherapy method, because it is my belief, after all I have proven, that it is the only method that works effectively and safely by encouraging a process in the body that promotes self-healing.

"Bioenergy therapy works, regardless of how it is performed" were the words of one biotherapist, when he gave a statement to a magazine. On the contrary, it matters significantly what method of biotherapy is applied. Methods do not "work" just because someone laid hands on you. And those hands as they say will "emanate" the cure, because that person has the "power" in their hands.

It is quite the opposite. It is not about any kind of "power" that someone claims to have or about any miracle. Pay close attention to who you will decide to go to for a treatment of bioenergy therapy. It is similar with any kind of other therapies. The contact should be established between you and the healer, whether they are a biotherapist, a doctor or a dentist. I was writing about the rule of the rapport in the Chapter 5. Without rapport, none of the therapy will work, or at least it will not work in a good way.

There are conditions for which treatment of biotherapy is not applicable:

- All types of emergency treatment
- Anaphylactic shock
- Extra-uterine pregnancy
- Appendicitis

The only good and proper explanation of how Biotherapy works is that scalar waves are forcing the cells of the body of the person that is receiving treatment to return to a healthy state, reversing the time of the disease.

It is quite understandable that it is better if the bioenergy therapy occurs in the early stages of the disease, when the disease has not progressed very far. Thus tissues of the body are still preserved, and there has been no massive degradation or destruction of cells. Biotherapy is also a very good addition to and support of medical therapy. Biotherapy never eliminates medical therapy and should never be used exclusively in place of recommended medical therapy. And although the decision is yours alone, and it is up to you how you will overcome your illness, do not ignore to include a high quality biotherapy.

In making your decision, it will surely help you to know that a positive mental approach towards your disease is necessary for effective healing and you should not just treat the symptoms.

A good example for that is a treatment for headache. It is definitely a daily problem of millions of people in all forms of intensity, from weak to severe. When we take a pill for a headache, we are treating the symptom. Pain is a symptom. Pain tells us that something is wrong. And we usually do not know what the cause of the pain is until some other signs of disease or disorder occurs. Headaches can be a symptom of many diseases. One of the causes of a headache is commonly known and very dangerous. It is stress. Stress is not a disease, but it certainly leads to it. The disease affects us long before we are able to perceive any signs of it.

Our Aura shows damage long before the disease is noticed, and it is only a matter of time before the disease appears in full swing on the physical body.

When, how and in which part of the body the disease is going to present itself depends on the person and the strength of her or his immune system. Another factor is how well the bioenergy flows through the energy centers or chakras in the whole human body.

There is no state of perpetual health, and a truly healthy person does not exist. We are constantly exposed to a variety of pathogenic agents in our environment, and thus are exposed to all kind of diseases.

There are very significant differences that can be observed in the course of a disease and its recovery. A person, whose bioenergy in the body is in balance, shows a significantly shorter time in suffering or recovering from illness.

A major part in the treatment of the individual is ones willpower to be healed. Bioenergy therapy is influenced by the willpower and determination to improve healing. A person's will is not measurable, nor can it be displayed. But disease can easily weaken the willpower of the individual. Only when the patient realizes that he is doing better is when he comes to the realization that her or his willpower was seriously compromised. For many patients the very first contact with the bioenergy therapy method is initially to learn that it is possible to heal themselves, and that a human being is, to a large extent, more than just a physical body that has failed.

When disease happens, it is logical that the individual requests medical assistance. From that moment on, their life has a whole new rhythm and rules, and everything will begin to revolve around how many drugs they will have to consume, when the next doctor's appointment is going to take place, and fear of what they will hear about the state of their health, i.e. about their disease, during that doctor visit. This is a tremendous amount of thinking that must be held at bay to control the disease.

When a patient comes in for a bioenergy therapy, he is neither able nor willing to accept the vicious cycle of drugs and visits to the doctor's office. But, however, it has been proven that such patients, even after just a few days of therapy, feel the change in themselves and their view of the disease. They are coming out from the narrow framework of their medical therapy and are beginning to realize that the only obstacle to a framework that hurtled their thoughts to spin in a circle were they alone. Not only will their view of the disease change, but also their whole life will change. *They leave their first bioenergy therapy with the knowledge that there is a bioenergy, which is available to all of us, and that they will be able to be cured.* These people are getting a whole new world and a new lease on life. Often, after coming to this realization nothing is as it was before.

Patients, who are for the first time attending a bioenergy therapy, come away with hope, disbelief, or a mixture of both emotions. It is particularly important to establish contact with the patient and bring them into the so-called medial condition. The term medial condition could be described as an alert, relaxed state, which I have described in previous chapters as the Field of Positive Intentions. If you would ultimately like to express it in some units of measurement, it is precisely the state of brain waves in the frequency of 7-13 Hz. This means that ideally speaking brainwaves are in the Alpha frequency. How can we reach this stage?

The therapy takes place either in a group or in individual sessions. Both ways of treatment are having their own advantages.

If the patient wants to be alone with the healer, her or his wish should be respected.

However, being in the group setting has many advantages. Treatment in a large group setting is recommended to the patients because the positive energy in this area is very strong, intense and concentrated. The patients, that are sitting and waiting for their turn, take advantage of the intense energy fields in the room and some are even remaining after their treatment. The entire group benefits from this energy even when they are not in direct treatment. It is also beneficial for the entire group to see the success and improvements of the others. That way they can assure themselves and see with their own eyes that the method works. The assurance and certainty that the method works is not going in the favor of the healer, it is going in the favor of the patient. He sees firsthand that the method works for everyone, and that it is just a matter of time before he himself will experience the improvement. The patient thus acquires a positive state of mind that is medial and has a Positive Field of Intent. It is one of the most important effects that almost 100% ensures the success of biotherapy. Biotherapy acts to stimulate the patient's body to heal itself, i.e. the cells are filled with bioenergy and are beginning to function normally.

We know that the improvement happens. We are conducting energy on the patient with the intention and commitment to heal. Some patients feel improvement almost immediately. If we do therapy because of pain of the bones or joints, after an operation or the like, then we are immediately asking the patient during and after the treatment if she or he feels improvement. Or we ask them to try to walk, if the problem was related to that part of the body.

In addition to the direct benefits of bioenergy performed on the patient, it is possible to successfully apply a distant bioenergy treatment. In doing so, the patient may be located thousands of kilometers away from the healer. Distance is not important, and the effect of therapy takes place in a split second. In this way, significant results are achieved in the treatment of sports injuries. In some treatments, the symptom of the disease can show relief and improvement toward healing on the fourth day of therapy, or a week after the first block of therapy of four days, or up to 3 months later.

Dealing with treatments of bioenergy, just like any other method of treatment involves basic knowledge of medicine, such as the layout and function of certain organs and their ailing conditions.

It is important to know that a person cannot apply Biotherapy to himself. It is not possible, because there must be an interaction of the energy field or aura between the two people, i.e. between the healer and the person that is receiving the therapy. It is the union and touching between the aura of the patient with the aura of the healer, and has nothing to do with taking or giving energy. The therapist or healer does not give any of his own energy to the patient. He is only conducting the energy from the space around us to the patient through his hands. The therapists serve as mediators and conductors.

This is, for the most part, the reason why the technique itself has to be learned practically in at least a group of two, and this is why the description of the method is impossible to be described in any book.

It is also important to know that the bioenergy therapists are not giving a diagnosis. Prior to any treatment, the therapist must have a medical diagnosis so that he will know precisely which treatments to perform. Therefore it is useful to emphasize once again that you should go to the doctor and try to find out what kind of disorder you have. The exception are those healers who are able to "read" the Aura, whether they are synesthetic persons or are in possession of knowledge and the GDV device by Prof. Korotkov. However, "reading" of an Aura is a science of its own, and I would advise all of you who are intending to be a healer, to concentrate yourself on your state of mind and where to learn the technique practically and profoundly.

The biotherapy treatment method is especially suitable for all problems of the mind and spirit, starting with daily sufferings, struggle and difficulties of the individual.

Maybe you have just decided to achieve a higher sense of quality into your life.

In some cases it is necessary to include medical Hypnosis therapy. In my office, I often treat the same patient with both types of therapy, bioenergy and medical Hypnosis. Of course, in any case, not both at the same time.

A skillful bioenergy therapist will be able to help you no matter how big or small your steps towards progress and maintaining your health are.

It is well worth the effort to find a local bioenergy therapist. I am sure you will find one because the number of qualified therapists is becoming more prevalent

For more information on choosing a bioenergy therapist in your area or region of the world you can contact us by contacting us through our website: www.bioenergy-balance.com or www.bioenergieheilung.ch

Medical Hypnosis Therapy

Hypnosis is a method and a type of the holistic therapy that is very effective. However it has nothing in common with any magic. In spite of this, Medical Hypnosis cannot treat all medical conditions. But with those areas that Medical Hypnosis can treat, it is very effective, and sometimes even more successful than some other methods. In some cases, hypnosis is used to make a person open in communicating with other people and their environment in a way that it opens up a person toward himself. This opens up a whole range of features and a completely new mental picture and horizons.

For better understanding, and to erasing the doubt, I am giving you herewith a few facts from scientific research on hypnosis as a method of medical treatment:

EEG measurements (encephalographic), meaning the images of the brains electrical current, have shown that the EEG of the person under hypnosis is almost the same as that of a person's EEG that is fully awake. This means that there is no unconscious or unaware state of mind in which the patient does not know what's going on with him or her. Brainwave frequencies range from between 5 Hz and 13 Hz, which mean that the state of hypnosis is conducted in a range of brain frequency of theta and alpha waves. The person, to which hypnosis treatment is applied, may voluntarily terminate a session.

The person is in a state that resembles strong relaxation, which is then reflected in quiet breathing and low blood pressure.

Contact between the hypnotherapist and the patient can be interrupted, in that the patient falls asleep during the hypnotic session, but he wakes up in a few minutes.

Hypnosis Therapy is never a kind of act of power or dominance of a therapist over the client in which the client loses control of himself. Supreme importance is to always have the relationship of confidence between the person receiving therapy and the hypnosis therapist.

This is the main and most important requirement which, if absent, excludes any possibility of therapy with the person concerned.

After a therapy has been completed, a person who has been inducted into the hypnosis is "coming back" in a way that the therapist would count numbers.

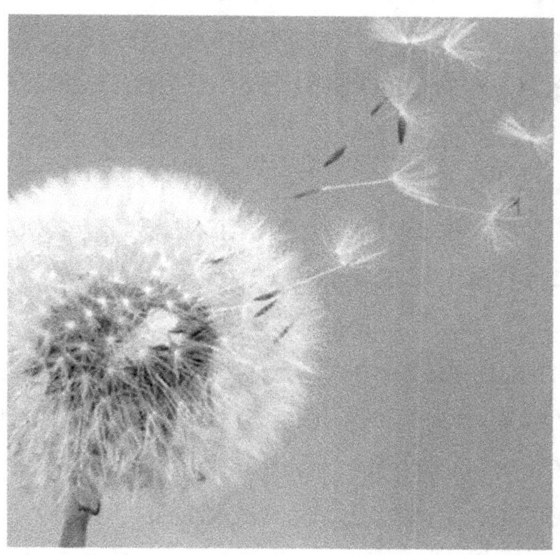

Hypnosis as a medical therapy has a wide application in a variety of branches such as:

Medicine: Allergies, heart diseases and diseases of circulatory systems, neurological disorders, disturbances in bowel habits, autoimmune disorders

(Morbus Crohn, colitis ulcerosa), gynecology, surgery (surgery without anesthesia).

Dentistry / Dental Medicine: A relaxation of the patient, relief from fear, overcoming pain and reduce the threshold of pain, controlling conditions like vomiting and irritability when working in the oral cavity, reducing bleeding in surgery, working with people with hemophilia, helping in adapting foreign body (dentures).

Sports: Fear of competition, optimizing of motor muscle movements, incorporating positive mental concepts and skills, overcoming pain and fear of being beaten.

Psychology: depression, burn out, anxiety disorders, all kinds of phobias, sleep disorders, posttraumatic conditions, disorders related to eating food (bulimia, anorexia nervosa), sexual problems, mania, cognitive learning disabilities, public speeches (papers, exams, management, applying for jobs, etc.), disturbances in speech, communication, neurosis, a condition caused by cancer and general weakness of the immune system, coping with stress, addictions (alcohol, smoking, eating).

Law and Order: In America, medical hypnosis is often applied in the court system for the purpose of questioning a witness or a victim, to overcome amnesia or memory loss, as well as to enable the inducement of the therapy for the victims due to domestic violence.

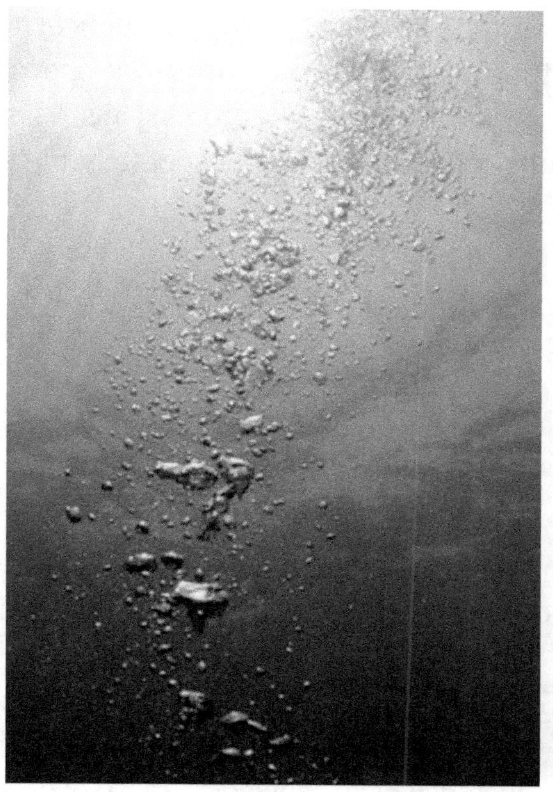

Milton Erickson, an undisputed expert in hypnosis, set the basic principles of modern hypnosis therapy. He believes that the people themselves are coming into a state of self-hypnosis, a light trance, several times a day, and that they are not aware of it.

Therapeutic group hypnosis is used as a highly successful method of achieving the goal of reducing body weight. Deep in the subconscious, hypnosis can motivate a person in such a way that the person creates a better self-image and achieves a more positive attitude in life. As a consequence, there is a positive thinking that is constructive as opposed to the situation in which a person is forcing his or her self to lose weight because they are desperately in need to do so.

Quitting smoking is very successfully treated by hypnosis therapy.

A scientific work conducted under the auspices of the Smoke International Organization showed a 95% success rate of abandoning smoking by people who undergo hypnosis treatment in combination with therapy called Neuro Lingual Programming (NLP).

In the Scientific Center at the School of Medicine at Texas A & M University, a study of clinical hypnosis has been conducted which showed that 81% of all people who have undergone the hypnosis therapy permanently terminated their smoking habit.

This is a chance for those who really want to quit smoking, and have tried various methods without success. If you are also belonging to that group of people, you may try hypnosis therapy. It is certainly worth trying.

Application of Clinical Medical Hypnosis in Psychoneuroimmunology

In addition to various psychological conditions, which are the essential causes of many medical disorders and even serious diseases, clinical medical hypnosis has a highly positive effect on the brains electrical currents, leading to brain activity with frequencies that are improving the patient's self-healing of his body. This is the main subject and topic of the Psychoneuroimmunology, which, as the newest branch of neurology, has led to spectacular new discoveries in medicine and is the subject of intensive scientific studies and experiments around the world.

How does it work in a simple terms?

If a person is burdened with thoughts that rotate around one topic, which is linked to an event that has happened previously, similar to what I described at the beginning of the book, it sometimes happens that the person is not able to resolve and get rid of these kinds of thoughts, which are consequently damaging the whole body. Even if the person has the necessary basic knowledge, so that she or he can otherwise help himself or herself, there are situations where they cannot get rid of the thoughts.

Thoughts are spinning in their heads and are beginning to create a vicious cycle so that this person alone is not able to free their self and should seek professional assistance. The most effective way, and probably the only possible way, is to implement medical and clinical applied hypnosis therapy.

Such a burden of bad thoughts is essentially nothing but undesirable resonances in the brain of the person concerned. The more one tries to get rid of these thoughts and to kick them out of his head, the more that the undesirable thoughts are spinning in a circle, constantly returning to the same subject. The mind is multiplying all kind of related thoughts in your head, as if it would glide through an imaginary spiral funnel, deeper and deeper, being ingrained in the subconscious.

Such bad thoughts or undesirable resonances cannot be "ejected" from someone's head. They must be replaced by other resonances. Otherwise, we will have the bad and undesirable resonances affecting our body cells, giving them information through the neurons in the brain that would be harmful. These are the prerequisites for an unrestricted way toward disease.

Briefly, you can say for hypnosis, that this is a phenomenon, which is shaping a better future for a person who has undergone a hypnosis therapy. In matter of fact it is a benefit to all mankind.

Jin Shin Jyutsu[R]

What must be understood from the very beginning about any kind of science is the basic premise of what the science can accomplish. The quintessence of the treatment is to understand from the beginning that no one can heal us as well as we can heal ourselves. Our body heals itself.

What is Jin Shin Jyutsu?

Jin Shin Jyutsu is the science and technique of effective treatments that accesses energy from our hands. It is based on bioenergy, which has been enabled to flow smoothly through the body. It is at the same time a fitness for the body, mind and spirit, simultaneously.

History of Jin Shin Jyutsu

Beneficial effects of the healing by hand techniques are known and have been used for millennia by various cultures, many of which have been forgotten until they were awakened from oblivion in the early 20th century.
The founder of Jin Shin Jyutsu, **Jiro Murai,** is a Japanese man who was born to a rich doctor in 1886, and was living a pretty lighthearted life. He was a young man who often overindulged in food and pizza, and got seriously ill at the age of 26. After the medical treatments became hopeless, he began to work

intensively in the art of healing based on the old masters, their techniques and meditations. He was especially interested in the healing of laying of the hands or fingers on specific points on the body that are responsible for the passage of bioenergy as well as various positions of the fingers, which are called *Mudras*. After he learned about the method and having healed himself, he devoted himself to the study of human diseases and the methods of treating them through the hands and fingers.

As a language interpreter, **Mary Burmeister,** an American lady of Japanese descent who was born in 1918 in the USA, met Master Jiro Murai during a visit in Japan. As Jiro Murai asked her whether she wanted him to teach her a technique of a healing treatment, she answered laconically with "yes", without knowing that this would change her whole life. Mary Burmeister learned the art of healing with hands and fingers from Jiro Murai over the next 12 years. She practiced intensely and began teaching the techniques in America for the first time in 1963, two years after the death of Master Jiro Murai. Mary Burmeister became a proponent of the Jin Shin Jyutsu philosophy. Until her death in 2008 she lived in Scottsdale, Arizona. Today there are therapists of Jin Shin Jyutsu in more than 20 countries around the world. Her family has licensed the method.

Alice Burmeister with Tom Monte: "The Touch of Healing; Energizing Body, Mind and Spirit with the Art of Jin Shin Jyutsu "(1997)

Differences between Jin Shin Jyutsu and Reiki

There are other treatment techniques and therapies that are based on the same principle of an undisturbed flow of bioenergy through the body. However they work with other principles and symbols. One such technique is, for example, *Reiki.* I mention it only as a comparison towards Jin Shin Jyutsu, because I have never studied it and have not tried it myself, so therefore I will not go into any description of Reiki techniques.

Reiki is also like Jin Shin Jyutsu in that it is also a Japanese healing technique. While Reiki works with chakras and symbols, it is only applied through the assistance of a skilled master of Reiki, which activates the flow of bioenergy in the chakras. In Jin Shin Jyutsu there are 26 energy points on the body, through which the blockages that are caused by many diseases and illnesses of the mind and body can be released. This is happening because Bioenergy cannot freely circulate. In difference to Reiki, the technique of Jin Shin Jyutsu can be performed by anyone, whether on himself or on others, with some basic prior knowledge and exercise.
Jin Shin Jyutsu is a healing art that influences the body, mind and spirit, and therefore incorporates therapeutic techniques, physiology, psychology and philosophy all

at the same time.

Benefits of treatment by Jin Shin Jyutsu

I will briefly present the methods of the treatment technique called Jin Shin Jyutsu because I have learned to apply this technique on myself during the course of my self-treatment. Later I have applied it on other people as well.

There are a lot of benefits, and side effects of these techniques do not exist. One should not cancel their appointment with their medical doctor because Jin Shin Jyutsu cannot replace medical diagnosis and treatment by conventional medicine. But it can significantly complement the conventional medicine.

Treatment using the Jin Shin Jyutsu method can be applied yourself if you need immediate help. The method is free, brings the balance of the body to a higher level, prevents the possible development of the disease, increases self-confidence and helps you to better understand yourself and the healing process. Therefore it is recommended as the support technique to the other therapies. This technique of bioenergy healing harmonizes the whole body with a goal to balance the body, mind and spirit. This is a healing Method you can perform anywhere and anytime. The method of Jin Shin Jyutsu has no harmful side effects or consequences.

But...
In cases of severe diseases, chronic fatigue or distraction and pain appearing repeatedly, there is an urgent need to take a therapy by a skilled therapist of Jin Shin Jyutsu who will be able to determine the exact position and be effective on certain points on the body in a way that the blockage of the flow of energy can be removed.

How the Jin Shin Jyutsu technique works

The Jin Shin Jyutsu technique is based on the fact that the body, mind and spirit are unique. Therefore this technique is helping a person, not only just in one of these three areas, but is interactive in all three, and this is because they are unique. This means that the technique helps both the body and the spiritual level in that it has a direct impact on them. As a result, this art of healing combines physiology, psychology and philosophy, simultaneously.

How is the Bioenergy in the body regulated by the Jin Shin Jyutsu technique?

The bioenergy method by Master Jiro Murai and the successor of his technique, Mary Burmeister, is spreading through the so-called "flow power gates" upon which there are 26 "locks" in the human body. Those are located on the front and back of the body. If a general imbalance or imbalance in the flow of bioenergy exists through one or more of the "power gates" or "energy locks", then that person is subjectively experiencing a state of discomfort or even illness.

During the flow of Bioenergy, our hands are comparable with the jumper cables in the car: the battery cables attached to the car that brings the energy to start the car. Our hands are performing the same by bringing the bioenergy to certain "energy locks" to the body.

The only difference compared to the human body energy is that a transfer of energy does not work almost immediately as the car starter, but it takes its effect after about 3 minutes.

Depending on the problem that is being treated in the body, treatment may take daily repetitions over several weeks. It depends on how many "energy locks" have been blocked, so that those will be brought to the point to be able to receive the energy again. Lying of the hands on specific points on the body is removing the blockage, so that the bioenergy can freely flow through the body.

Not only our hands, but also especially our fingers, can release blocked energy from specific "energy locks".

Fingers as the main driving techniques of Jin Shin Jyutsu

Your fingers cannot only touch the "energy points" on the body, release the barriers and facilitate the flow of bioenergy, but the fingers themselves are the holders of the energy points. Each of the fingers on our hand has several different energy points that are corresponding to the psychophysical structure of the body and thereby are having an impact on our body and spirit.

The awareness of one's self is the first step toward a treatment

The application of all bioenergy techniques, as well as of the Jin Shin Jyutsu technique, is having an impact on the mental balance of the person, as well.

The longer the Jin Shin Jyutsu technique is performed, the more the change is visible by each one of us, no matter if it is worry, fear, anger, and the way these emotions have an impact on us. Don't make yourself any illusions because this change will not happen overnight. But if you start today, and perform this method regularly, you will become aware that after some time your attitude towards things has changed, and you will start seeing things around you from a different perspective. This consequently means that your action and reaction will be significantly different from the earlier ones.

Start with it today and observe the changes - it's worth it.

What is the explanation of the term "Recognize Yourself"?

I will clarify this subject very briefly, for the knowledge of a person about himself is the main code for the very base of each treatment, whether you are healing yourself on your own or are having the treatment by a trained bioenergy therapist. You can decide, as well, to combine this treatment as a complementary treatment along with some therapy of conventional medicine.

Mudras - Finger fitness in the technique of Jin Shin Jyutsu

Mudras are gestures and symbols in Hinduism and Buddhism. Some of them include the entire body, but most are applicable to the hand gestures and fingers.
They are considered to be a specific energy stamp that is applied in the spiritual practice of religions and classical dances in India. Also, Mudras have been used in **Yoga** and in conjunction with breathing exercises in Yoga, Pranayama. This is practiced as part of some positions in yoga where we want to encourage the flow

of Prana, or energy, through the body.

Jiro Murai, founder of the Jin Shin Jyutsu technique, which is known today thanks to the work of Mrs. Mary Burmeister in the U.S., developed the positions of the fingers on both hands during his own difficult illness. So with his own self-treatment, the awakening and initiation of the Jin Shin Jyutsu technique was developed.

The next seven Mudras implement the process of relaxation of body and mind; giving a new strength, vitality and creativity to the lifestyle. Those Mudras are improving the flow of bioenergy and anyone who applies it will be able to feel better.

Mudra 1: For the improvement of the vitality and against fatigue and depression

This Mudra diminishes fatigue of body and mind in everyday life and reduces stress. It is also relieving existing worries, fears and anger.
How it works: Put your left hand in front of you so that thumb looks to the right side. Grasp the thumb, forefinger and middle finger of the left hand with your right hand, so that the thumb of your right hand is on the upper part of the left hand, and the other fingers of your right hand are on the palm side of the left hand - on the roots of the fingers. Repeat the same with the

other side after having one side held about 3 minutes.

Mudra 2: For good nerves

This Mudra calms us down and makes us feel satisfied and ready to face new challenges.
How it works: Turn the palm of your left hand outstretched toward you. Left thumb is turned to the left. Straddle the thumb and fingers of your right hand around your little finger and a ring finger of the left hand, so that the thumb of your right hand is in the front of you and the other fingers of your right hand are covering your left hand on the backside. Repeat the same with the other side and hold for 3 minutes.

Mudra 3: To solve and get rid of your burdens, to calm the mind, spirit and body. For the revitalization of all organs and their function. It is also reduces the need for sugar and sweets.

This Mudra helps us to get rid of frustrations, fears and everything that burdens us. It works well generally as well as specifically - which means, it allows us to get rid of a particular problem, or in general, you are able to ban the thoughts that haunt you throughout the day. It also reduces stress and leads to a better functioning of all organs.
How it works: with the middle finger and thumb of your right hand, straddle the outstretched thumb on

your left hand in such a way that the two fingers of your right hand are closing circuit. After doing that, place the nail on the tip of the thumb of the left hand. The thumb of your right hand is on the bottom side of your left hand thumb. Hold for 3 minutes and switch the hands.

Mudra 4: For relaxation of the back muscles and a general feeling of well-being

This Mudra will help you to breathe better and release the stiffness in your back muscles. Generally you'll feel better.
How it works: Click the nails of the middle fingers on both hands to one another. Hold for at least 3 minutes.

Mudra 5: For a good exhalation and releasing of tension in the head and lungs

This Mudra helps to relieve the tension of the head and lungs and a good exhaling in order to get rid of all those particles of dust and dirt that have accumulated in our body throughout the day while breathing the air.
How it works: Cross the fingers of both clasped hands except of the middle fingers that extend vertically.

Mudra 6: For easier and deeper breathing

This Mudra helps by difficulties with the ears. It decreases the pressure in the ears, so that it is recommended while flying or simply being on high altitudes. It also helps with problems with the skin.
How it works: Press the nail of the middle finger on the tip of the thumb of the same hand, so that two fingers are closing the circuit. Hold for 3 minutes.

Mudra 7: Against stress

This Mudra is a good help in all stress situations. It helps to relax.
How it works: Press the fingertips of the thumb and index finger closing the circuit. Hold on both hands for 3 minutes.

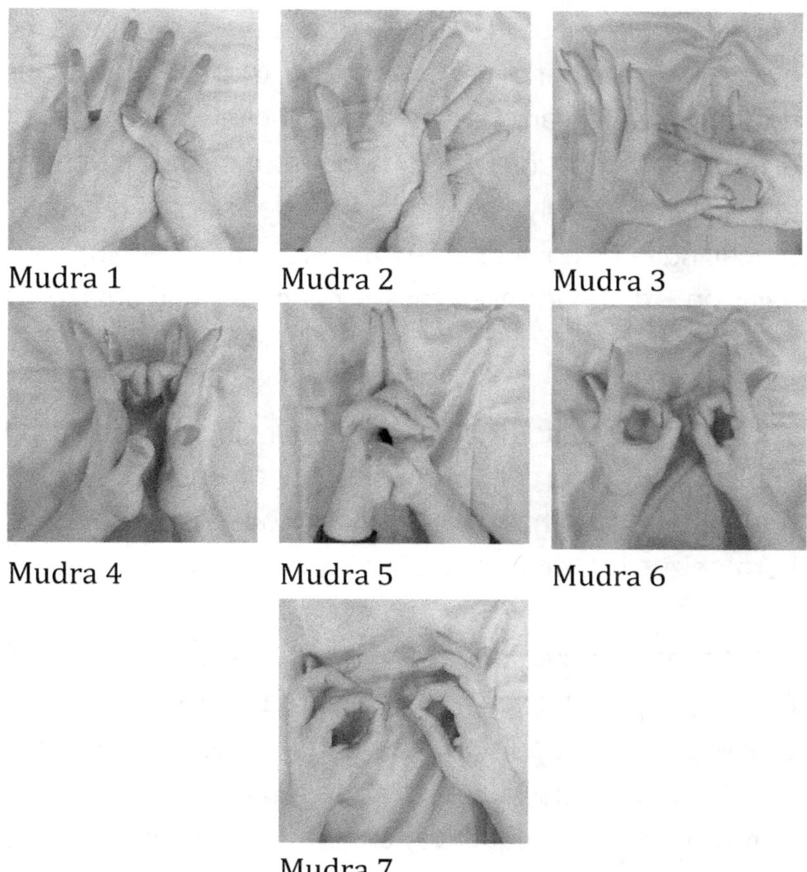

Mudra 1 Mudra 2 Mudra 3

Mudra 4 Mudra 5 Mudra 6

Mudra 7

The power of healing is in our fingers

By simply holding the fingers of one hand with the other, as if those would be the booster cables, helps to harmonize the energy of mind, body and spirit. It also represents one of the most important ways of "Self Aid".

Through this method we are reducing the effects of everyday stress and are influencing the change of our thoughts, which are as result, significantly affecting all of our body functions. Our thoughts can be influenced and changed only by our own decision. The daily practicing of holding the fingers can deepen our decision to undertake these changes and make it happen.

The simple technique of holding your fingers should be applied daily in order to enable flow of energy through the body, so that it remains constant and thus harmonizes the mind with all body functions.

We distinguish five basic patterns that are creating and forming our thinking. These are fear, anxiety, anger, sadness and compulsion (pushing yourself due to lack of satisfaction). This creates certain models of thoughts that are, as a consequence, creating our opinions about something. If these 5 basic principles are repeating, then we are trapped in those and are spinning around in a circle between certain patterns of thinking (fear, anxiety, anger, sadness or compulsion) and the consequences of such an attitude. Here is an example: often we are faced with something that is new, and as a result we have a fear of being unsuccessful and becoming unsafe, which automatically creates an even greater fear. If we, however, as a child through the age of 4, have received a positive feedback from our environment as well as encouragement, then as adults, we will stay attracted to new developments and will respond with curiosity and with self-confidence.

Models for all subsequent reactions and the world of man's thoughts are formed till the age of 4. Those children who did not get this kind of support from their surroundings are as adults having problems to cope with everyday life.

In using our thoughts, we are creating our own world. The source of our thoughts is in harmony when they are not dominating us. Instead of that there is an inner peace and harmony. One should not have big emotional leaps between wild elation and excessive expectations and fear. Our soul is at peace. In this state we are open to receive the message of the Creator.

Through daily finger exercises, we are achieving deep-rooted attitudes, which can capture our minds.

Jiro Murai and Mary Burmeister found that in each finger of our hands, there are different energy flows, which can affect our mood, attitudes, thoughts and functions of the body.

The time and place of the daily finger exercises, as well

as the order in which grasp the finger of one hand with the other hand has no significance.

Holding the thumb keeps us free of worry

If you think about it, you will find that you cannot change what has happened yesterday, and that what will be tomorrow has not happened yet. Therefore, the only moment in which we find ourselves is the here and now. The only power that can be used creatively is the one you do not waste away, but are using at the present moment.

Holding our thumb regularly every day relieves worries, fears, and obsession of certain thoughts, along with feelings of hatred and depression. It works extremely well on the function of the stomach and spleen, helping us to find a balance in the middle of our bodies. A feeling of heaviness or even being sick to your stomach if you are worried is well known.

Holding the forefinger liberates us from fear

This grip helps us to get rid of fear, insecurity and perfectionism. People who are free of fear and are carrying within themselves the feeling of satisfaction promote the work of the immune system, and are thus contributing to the treatment of diseases. This was confirmed by recent immunological studies.

Holding the index finger helps the function of the kidneys and bladder. It has been known for a long time that fear can affect the emptying of the bladder.

If you are in the dentist's office, hold your index finger with your other hand. You will realize that the fear is being suppressed.

Holding the middle finger frees us from rage.

When our day is full of frustration and anxiety, and things have not gone as intended, or if aggressive behavior is part of our everyday life, holding the middle finger helps us to break free of that frustration. Anger is actually amassed creative energy, which then can be released towards the person opposite of us, and most possibly towards the wrong person. Holding the middle finger helps us to use this kind of creative energy so that it indeed serves creativity.

In reference to the associated organs, the middle finger covers the function of the liver and bile. Probably everyone knows the saying: "This or that is getting on my liver."

Holding the ring finger liberates us from sorrows.

Holding our ring finger helps us to let the things go and allow us to separate ourselves from them. Whether it is the clothing that has accumulated in the closet or it is a friendship that is for us no longer appropriate.

To branch out and let something go, especially let go of someone, means to say goodbye and to go through a grieving process. It helps people who are unable to mourn or cry, which is a very important process of making peace within themselves. In addition, the holding of the ring finger helps harmonize guilt and make it easier to overcome such states of mind. We know deep within us that the current situation is temporary and that we will see better times. Be aware that when we are in difficulties, it helps us get through this situation.

In reference to the associated organs, holding the ring finger helps the lung and colon function, releasing the free flow of energy. The impact on the colon is in terms of enhanced peristaltic.

Holding of the little finger

Holding your little finger should liberate you from stress that has arisen because of your efforts to perform certain tasks successfully that you do not like.

If we do not love what we do, it costs us a lot of effort and energy to overcome the uneasy feeling that is being generated, and we are investing significant energy and effort to do the job. The same situation happens with emotions. We are laughing on the outside but we are crying deep inside of our soul. There is a common saying: "That Hurts My Soul".

Holding the little finger helps us to feel at ease and stay truthful to our own values. And our life suddenly becomes easier. If we are living in a partnership, it is having a positive impact on our relationship as well.

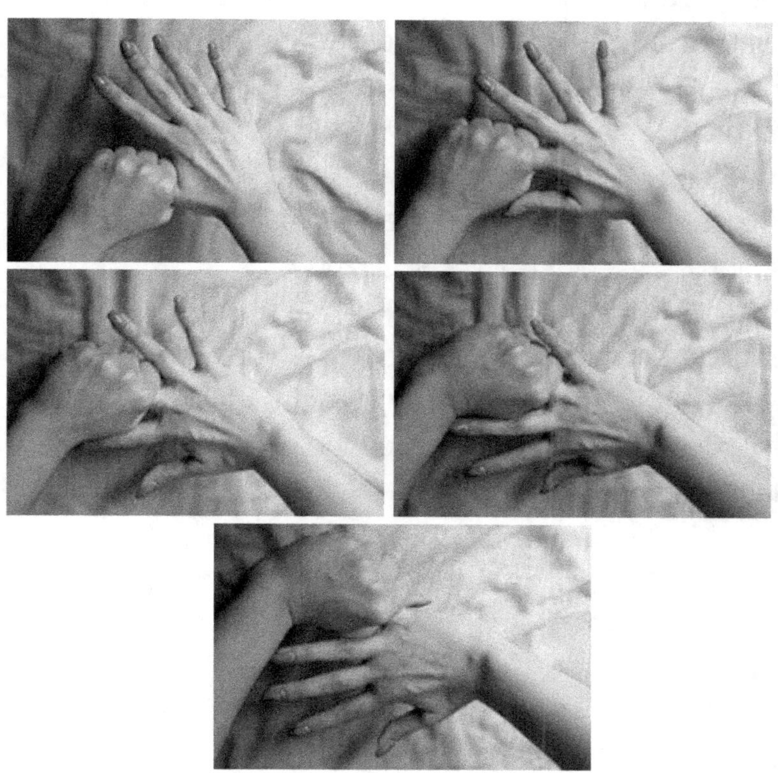

In reference to the associated organs, holding the little

finger harmonizes the energy of the heart and the area of the small intestine.

Jin Shin Jyutsu is immeasurably more than is offered here. We have only touched the very basics of the method. I hope that by describing this method in the simplest way the principles of these techniques will be of practical help to you.

New scientific research has proven that the same gestures and words are absorbed in the brain through bioenergy, leaving a kind of a seal in certain areas of the brain.

"Words, Gestures Are Translated By Same Brain Regions," Science Daily, 09.11.2000

Worth mentioning in the group of bioenergy therapies is also **Thai Yoga Therapy**, which is a 2500 year old discipline of traditional therapeutic treatment in Chinese Medicine and **Ayurveda**.

Thai Yoga Therapy

The Buddha himself, in collaboration with his personal physician Shivago Komarpaj, has developed Thai Yoga. It was designed as a practical application of the "Metta" state, which is the practice of love and kindness in Buddhism.

In practice, Thai Yoga is really a system of physical meditation that has the task and function to stimulate the flow of bioenergy or prana in a way that the acupressure points of each Chakra are targeted.

Nuad Bo - Barn, meaning "touch of ancient healing", was a 2,500 thousand year-old form of Thai Yoga that has been developed under the strong influence of Yoga and Buddhism as well as traditional methods of treatment, such as Ayurveda and elements of Chinese medicine.
In its structure, the technique is based on the theory of Sen-lines, which are related to Nadis in Ayurveda.

The technique of Thai Yoga Therapy begins with the treatment of the feet and moving up the body to the head. It is a combination of techniques such as Trigger Point Treatment, Deep Pressure, and Restorative Yoga Postures i.e. beneficial Yoga Positions, to achieve relaxation.

Thai Yoga Therapy is widely usable, taking into account the age, the constitution and state of health of the person because its strength can be very deep or mild, depending on the client's needs.

In this way it is possible to therapy the people of most different conditions. Thai Yoga Therapy is an absolutely flexible discipline of bioenergy therapy.

Thai Yoga Therapy works by rising and improves lymphatic system entities, lowers blood pressure by bringing into balance and harmony the energetic and spiritual components.

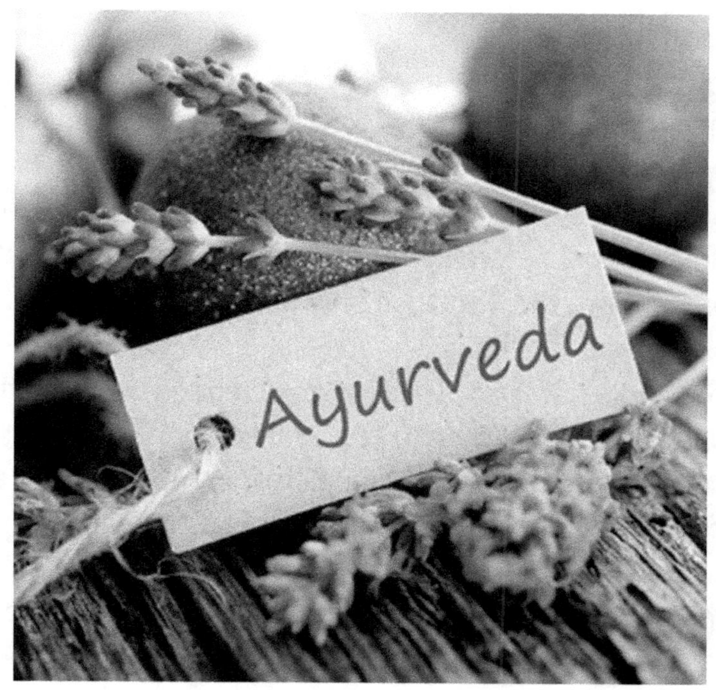

Ayurveda

The earliest reports of Ayurveda are found in the records of the Vedas. Vedas are the oldest tradition of the origin and concept of a human being and the universe, and are presenting universal laws of life, and were passed on verbally. These concepts were written in the language and script of Hinduism - Sanskrit. These records are contained in four books. Originally, the reports were passed verbally from generation to generation for thousands of years. It is believed that they were transferred to the Vedas in the period between 1200 B.C. and 700 B.C. in written form in the

Sanskrit language.

The word Veda in translation means knowledge.

It is said that the knowledge contained in the Vedas is endless and eternal, and that human knowledge, compared to the Vedas, is only a handful of dirt.

The studies that are tracking Ayurveda in Sanskrit from approximately 1000 B.C. reveal an astonishing knowledge of general medicine. Ayurveda is also described as the science of life and practiced from India to Nepal and Sri Lanka. As Buddhism flourished in the 6th century B.C., Ayurveda has been passed on through the Buddhist priests to Tibet, China and Mongolia, where it remained until today.

One of the records of Ayurveda, which also dates from the same period, i.e. 1000 years B.C., Susruta Samhita, was relatively recently translated into German. In particular this record was the basis for the beginning of the development of today's modern plastic surgery.

Essential recognizable AUMmmm mystical sounds were used in many Dharma religions, such as Hinduism, Buddhism, Sikhism and Jainism. In the Upanishads it is written: "It is the highest form of support. Whoever knows only that single one mystical sound, gets everything he wants."

In simple terms, Ayurveda is a holistic system that has only one goal, which is to be a guideline for a healthier, and more balanced lifestyle. Ayurveda recognizes and respects the principles of the unique quality of every human being as an individual, basing their study on nutrition, yoga, massage and herbal preparations. The study and science of Ayurveda is a tribute to the uniqueness of life and is closely connected and united with the physical form of a human being as well as his mental and psychological aspects.

Ayurveda helps to achieve harmony and balance in all three aspects of the human being: physical, mental and spiritual. In this way it also helps generally human health, but also prevents the signs of aging by individuals.

Nutrition has an enormous impact on the entire human body, and if it is not balanced, it is leading to disease. But it's also a holistic approach to Ayurveda and its rules about the way of life responsible for the fact that where they have been applied and adopted, the treatments have successfully healed about 50% of all diseases. In many chronic and serious diseases is recommended to combine conventional medicine and Ayurveda.

It should never be forgotten that if you are ill and

decide to apply Ayurveda as your treatment and therapy, you should contact both of the experts of general medicine and Ayurveda.

What is the human reality and how it is created?

Divisions of the Vedas, called Rishas, are talking about the mechanism of projection. Projection is a mechanism by which human consciousness creates reality.
The best example of this is in the world of movies: the actors are projecting characters that act on to the consciousness of the viewer to create the impression of reality.

What we think becomes our reality.

Projections are building and creating opinions. The events themselves are totally insignificant, no matter what kind of event it is about. And they stay insignificant as long as we do not allow them to be significant.

"How many are the fires, how many suns, how many dawns, how many waters?
I address you o Pitris (ancestor), not for the sake of disputation; I ask you in order to know (the truth). "
(10.88.18) Veda

For more about the basics on the science of Ayurveda, which will help you to look for a healthy lifestyle, you should also read my book "How to Stay Healthy With Ayurveda".

Chapter 8

Holistic Sports

The opinion that sport and exercise of the body only has an importance in burning calories is deep-rooted. This is of course true, but the other remaining positive aspects are pushed far into the background. Although talking about sports has become very popular, and the general opinion is that if someone has a common general knowledge about physical activities then they believe they have an entire knowledge. However, the most recent scientific minds have found some details still unknown to the general public.

If we talk about fitness, then the notion of being "fit" has a meaning of being full of vitality, full of enthusiasm and energy. It is contained in the word fitness. To be engaged in fitness means to become and stay fit. But it also means to be well trained, mobile, and have a good shape, as well as to own a big advantage at the level of the body's cells. People engaged in fitness or any other physical activities have a greater number of mitochondria within their body cells.

Mitochondria are the organelle (something like "little organs"), which contain a very important enzyme. The effect of these enzymes is that they are actively involved in the creation of aerobic energy. The description of these enzymes can usually be found under the name "cellular exchangers of energy" because they produce energy by drawing it from the food we consume.

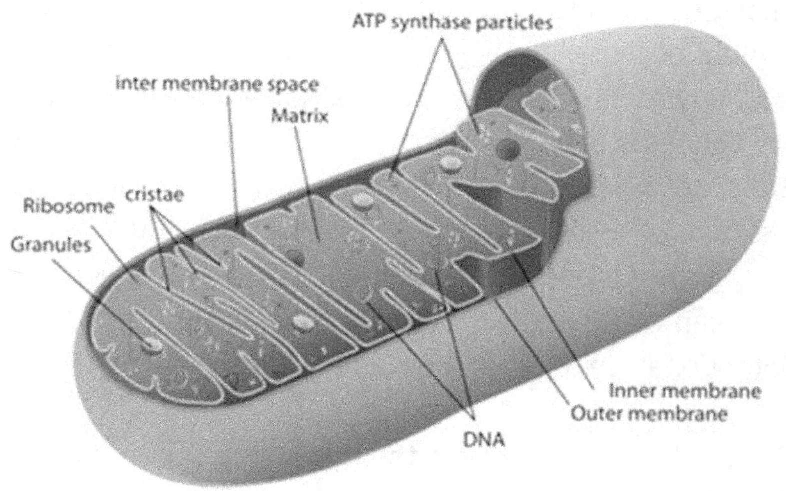

Why do we burn more calories when exercising or participating in any kind of sport? We are burning more calories because mitochondria also participate in the aerobic combustion of fatty acids, which is, simply put, the burning of fat in the body. This process also takes place when we are resting or sleeping.

The result of growth in the number of mitochondria

through exercise and physical activity is also boosting the metabolism so that it burns more calories. This process flows during exercise, but most of all when we have more rest and are not physically active.

Exercises in the field of physical fitness activities increase your strength and endurance. This has the consequence that you are able to do many activities more frequently than you would otherwise have done, simply because all of a sudden it is not as difficult for you anymore. And other physical activities are available to you as a possibility, because the more you realize that it can be done, the more you are performing these tasks with ease. This, in turn, is accumulating an energy level, one's self-confidence or belief in yourself, and can help with the situation in which you are on an intentional weight loss program.

It can happen suddenly that you stop losing weight. This is the so called Plateau which is a sudden halt of losing your weight, even as you continue to apply the same methods, workouts and diets that had previously functioned.

Types of sports that have a distinct component of bioenergy in an oriental tradition include **Thai Chi** and **Pilates.**

But it is up to you to choose the kind of sport and

physical activity that suits you. It can be Yoga, boxing, cycling, spinning, fencing, running on a treadmill, Thai Chi, Pilates or just brisk walking.

The positive effects of sport and physical activity in general on the body and mind of an individual are an indisputable fact. Sport is for everyone and there is no age limit. There is only a choice that fits your needs and situation, whether it is the purpose of your workouts, impact sports or low impact sport, benefits that you desire, how expensive the sport is or just your personal preferences. Everything is there for all people.

I would like to put the effect of sports on stress reduction in the most important place. Stress cannot be visible on the physical body. At least not right away. When it becomes noticeable, it is mostly too late. Of course concern must be taken in any sport and weigh the benefits of sport on the body.

An important effect of sport is the effect it has on our skin, whether it is a young person who has a problem with acne, or an older person with losses of collagen and disappearance of elasticity in the skin. Sweating in sport helps open the pores and cleanses the skin, as well as support of the muscles and its activity will enhance skin elasticity. Sport improves breathing, and thus the supply of oxygen increases in the entire body and the blood supply of the cells. The next benefit is that it affects the mobility and movability of a person, their joint mobility, bone structure and the whole skeleton, setup and balance of the spine, the support of all the muscles, glands of internal and external secretion, blood circulation, lymphatic flow and the coordination of movement and balance of a person.

Choose any kind of sport but just choose something.

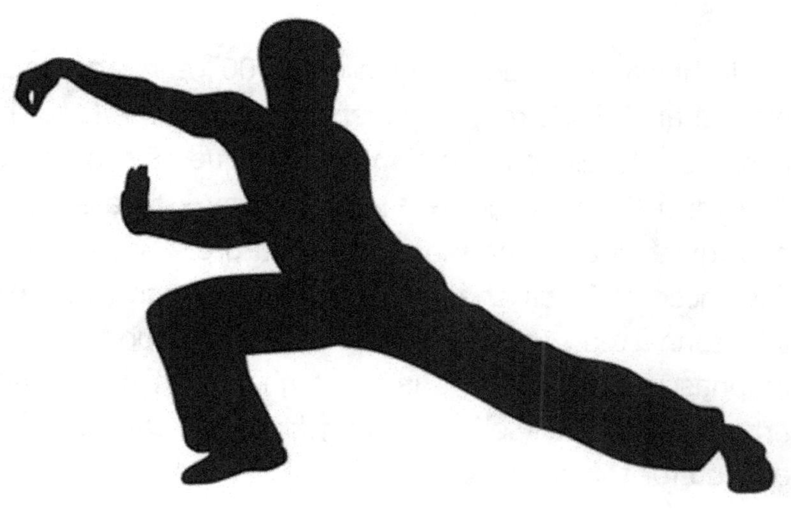

Thai Chi

Thai Chi is a type of sports activity that combines a lot of features and many benefits for all people. Thai Chi, which I am also practicing, would be described most appropriately as a kind of meditation in motion.

The advantage of this sport or exercise is that there is no age limit, physical boundaries or barriers. Anyone can be engaged in this sport activity. The concept of this sport is very simple, and has evolved into a graceful form of exercise. It comprises a sequence of movements implemented in a slow, focused manner and supplemented by deep breathing. It works for a person in a subtle way on a level of the bioenergy, or life force, for a person who performs it.

Thai Chi was initiated in China over 700 years ago as a martial arts skill strongly influenced by Taoism. Later it has been developed into a mild technique of exercises. The term "Tao" means - a path, a way - to a simple and quiet life in harmony with nature. Taoists are convinced that all the elements in the universe are interconnected and intertwined. It is important to emphasize that Thai Chi is the higher form of martial arts: it is not in itself a fighting skill, but can also be applied for this purpose.

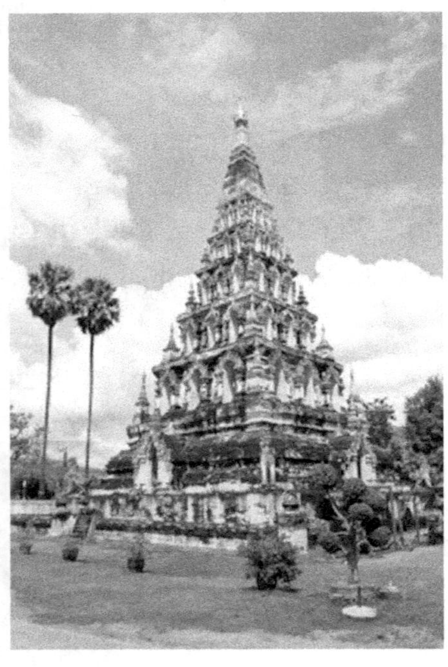

Translated Thai Chi means "supreme ultimate" and is commonly associated with a physical principle of "centering". This means that, in case of conflict, the goal is to merge the spirit and body in the center of the body.

The Tai Chi technique of exercises are slow running movements that seem to be transformed from one to the other, while maintaining the balance of the body by tilt, which greatly improves the strength in your legs, but also your balance. The person who performs these exercises is fully aware of his body as well of the position in which the body is located.

Results have been verified that this significant bioenergetics sport will assist in improving immunity and an improved mood. Medical practitioners have recognized that Thai Chi as a sport has benefits in health improvement and are recommending it as such.

One of my patients asked me, what must be done to get stress completely thrown out of his life. I answered that it was not possible, because life is stress. Instead of seeking a tool that will "destroy" the stress, it is better to seek and find the causes of stress, which can then be mitigated, prevented and kept under control.

It is also possible to target the reduction of stress and use a combination of methods of the physical, mental and psychological constitution of the individual, in order to hold back the effects of stress and anticipating in reducing it to a minimum.

It is scientifically proven that if our mind can be controlled so that the person is awake but in a very calm state of mind, the level of the stress hormone cortisol will significantly decrease. This will give a sense of peace and general satisfaction. At the same time it increases the number of cells in the body that have a positive effect on the immune system and thus of the entire organism.

Thai Chi is precisely that kind of sport and method that affects the body mind and spirit, and helps someone deal with stress positively. The effects of Thai Chi on stress reduction are medically proven.

Every detail in the technique of Tai Chi can be compared and transferred to the principles of Yin and Yang. Thai Chi is an exercise skill. Whoever participates in this sport is rewarded with increased mobility and balance, and even stronger breathing, a stronger lymphatic and blood system and reducing blood pressure.

The most effective way to learn Thai Chi is through a variety of books freely available worldwide. Nowadays quite a lot of information can be found on the Internet as well on the video sites available, such as YouTube. In this book I have strived to only introduce Tai Chi to you in a general outline, and you will find much more comprehensive books readily available. Hopefully this will give you the incentive to perhaps decide to enroll in a course of Thai Chi.

By that, I also want to emphasize, that in no case

should you decide to learn the technique and practice it only from videocassettes or books, because it's not possible. All movements in this sport, the inclination of the body, posture, breathing and coordination are so precise that to truly learn this method you should find a class. A good Tai Chi instructor can teach you the movements, and will correct your posture and breathing. In doing so, I suggest you choose a very experienced teacher. Thai Chi is at the same time a skill and an art.

If your doctor has recommended exercising with Thai Chi because of pain in the joints or for arthritis, as is often the case, consult with your doctor about the movements and your Thai Chi teachers about the condition of your joints. Never try to perform the movement by forcing yourself, especially when you feel that this movement is difficult to do. If you are not able to perform it, but you try to do it anyway, it could be damaging. If you exercise in the group lessons with others, do not be embarrassed if you do not do exactly the same posture and movement as a teacher or your classmates. Thai Chi is definitely a meditative technique, not an activity to create stress.

It is likely that you have seen a few scenes on television or film where the young and old are practicing together Thai Chi outdoors: in a very nice park, in the open air, or in nature. Quite often they are in China or some country in Asia and are employees of a company that promotes Tai Chi in the workplace. World trade is very competitive and many have paid a dear price not realizing what is happening to their employees. I had a patient who said that even then, when it happened, they did not notice the slightest sign that he ran into a "burn out". Large and small companies in China and Asia have implemented the practice of Tai Chi in their corporate logistics. It is optimal to exercise in a group, in the morning hours, in the fresh air. It not only has a positive effect on the employees, but also to the company itself.

The technique of Thai Chi consists of 24 exercises, which are movements that are flowing smoothly across each other.

Several factors have an impact on the exercise technique of Thai Chi. The first and most important effect is breathing and breathing techniques. It is important to become aware of breathing. First it starts with the body control. Chest and abdomen: the chest is flat to slightly indented, so that breathing is actually concentrated down to the stomach. In doing so you can sit or stand.

-**Relax** and begin to monitor your breathing in the spirit. You can at the same time close your eyes and

-**Focus** your mind - just by inhaling saying "breathe" in your mind, and by the exhalation saying, "exhale" in your mind.

-**Keep track of your body** - try to physically feel how the body runs out of breath during exhalation and fills up by inhalation.

-**Imagine** a balloon in the lower abdomen, which is filled with air and rises when you inhale, and vice versa, the balloon is empty, when you expire.

-**Feel** - place both hands on the lower abdomen and feel the balloon as it fills up and empties.

This breathing technique is unconditionally applied by exercising with Tai Chi, but you can apply it in case of stress in many situations as a separate breathing technique as well, which will put you in very short period of time in a relaxed mood and will reduce stress.

The next factor of the technique is the position of the waist and the pelvis, which must be relaxed and slightly recessed with both feet on the ground, knees slightly bent: a position that is comparable with the state of the body when riding.

Furthermore it is very important to distinguish between "empty" and "solid." It is a condition that occurs when the energy shifts in your feet through the legs: when the weight of the body switch to the left leg, it will become solid, and right leg will become empty and vice versa.

Arms, shoulders and elbows remain relaxed in a natural position.

All these factors affect the Thai Chi exercises so as to allow Chi or Bioenergy freely flowing through the body. Energy flow starts from the feet and legs rising over the waist and the shoulder to the hand and fingers.

People who choose the Thai Chi as their physical activity are also prone to a lesser degree to fall down as they get in a higher age and are having their body simply better under control.

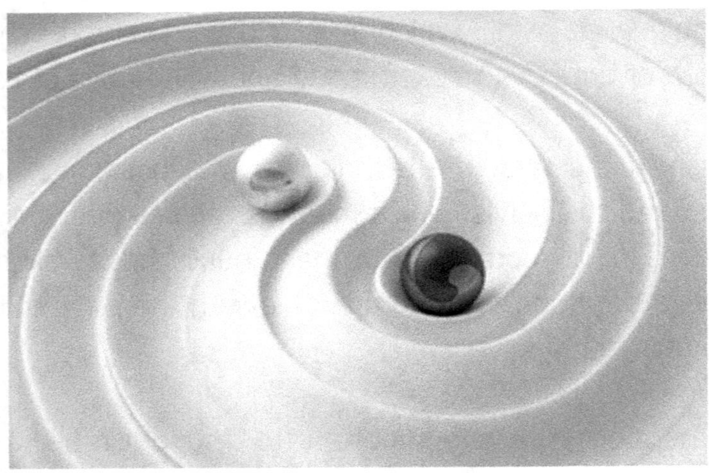

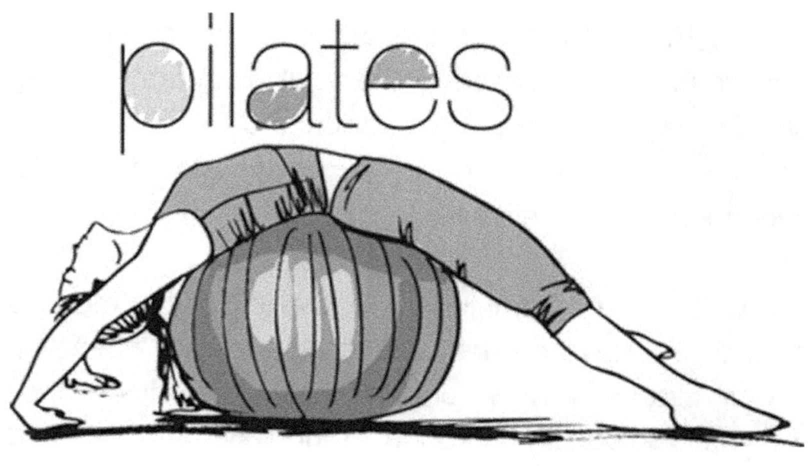

Pilates

Pilates is a complete fitness system, a specific group of physical exercises developed by Joseph Pilates in the early 20th century. Born in Germany in 1880 as a stunted and weak child suffering from asthma and rheumatic fever, Pilates was keen to strengthen his body and be healthier and more attractive. He started to do gymnastics and body building and, at the age of 14 years, posed for the pictures of the body in anatomy textbooks. These important details from the life of Joseph Pilates are quoted to show you that your goals in developing yourself physically are certainly possible. Maybe you can even see yourself and you find yourself in the same situation.

Pilates immigrated to England in 1912 and made a living demonstrating the methods of self-defense in the circus. His method was created primarily to help the recovering of wounded soldiers at the front during World War I, when he was stationed at a military base in Lancaster where he performed physiotherapy for wounded English soldiers.

In 1925 Pilates immigrated to the U.S. and met his future wife Clare on the boat to America. He opened a training studio in New York with her a year later, which he ran personally through 1960. He incorporated directly into his method that the mind controls the functioning of the muscles, and the muscles control the setup of the spine. The setup of the spine consequently controls the muscles of the chest, and these muscles, in order to further the chain, are working together with proper breathing control in the liberation of back and neck pain.

His first clients in the newly opened studio were professional dancers from Broadway, whose movements and flexibility were also incorporated into his training program.

In 2005, 11 million people were involved in the training of Pilates, only in USA.

The main objective of the creation and design of his exercise program is to establish a unification of the mind and body of a person who performs his exercises.

Pilates, as method of fitness, enables harmonization and balance of the body, mind and soul.

Pilate's exercises can be effective for you - no matter what your gender, age or physical condition. When you decide to practice Pilates, you must know that this method avoids any quick or sudden movements. Each movement is peaceful, but powerful, flexible, yet firm. Pilates helps strengthen the power and mobility of someone who exercises without increasing muscle mass.

The Pilates Method is based on the principles of centering, concentration, control, precision, breathing and fluid movement. It has a lot in common with yoga.

Centering in Pilates includes the abdomen; pelvis and gluteus that are called by a common name the "powerhouse" - a source of strength. It is the center and the crossing of all energies that are pouring in to this center and split again to the extremities, i.e. hands and feet.

Concentration and control are the connection between the minds controlling the muscles. So in the beginning of the development of his method, Pilates called his exercise program "Contrology", to emphasize the aspect of the direct influence of a mind on the muscles. The goal was to gain control of the mind as much as possible with more graceful movements, which are absolutely harmonized, and the number of movements is reduced to a minimum.

For this, more **precision** is required, which in practice can only be achieved by constant **control** of the movement.

Proper **breathing** is absolutely necessary in exercise to allow good circulation and optimum blood flow, which is a very important factor for the health of the body and acts on the cellular and organic level. In this way, not only cell function is improved, but also metabolism and rejection of harmful substances from the cells and organs. These harmful substances are causing fatigue, if they are not removed from the cells.

On the market, of course, you can get all kinds of literature, videos and DVDs of this popular method of exercise. They can serve as a support to be able to create the approach to the method visually. However, it is not advisable and even practically not possible to adopt a method of Pilates exercising by yourself without the help of a good trainer of the Pilates method.

A lot of factors that I enumerated earlier, operating simultaneously, must be controlled, and one person alone is not able to control all these aspects.

Pilate's exercises can be divided into two main groups: those that are performed on a mat and Pilate's exercises using exercise equipment.

Exercises on the mat are the most popular, easiest and little can be done to harm the person who performs it. Very often mats are utilized in exercise rehabilitation centers. The most important part of Pilates incorporates a good mat and extra hand elements such as large and small balls, and elastic bands. These elements, however, are not recommended in the initial phase of practicing Pilate's method.

Home sweet home. It is well known motto worldwide. There are many DVD's and videos on the market that will give you training on Pilates. But I recommend that you learn some basics through the videos, and then attend a Pilate's studio to learn more specific techniques with feedback from your instructors. There is no reason not to choose a Pilates exercise as your type of physical activity and practice it at home. By learning the principles you can then safely practice it at home. With no additional costs and large space. And without risk to get injured practicing.

Pilate's exercises are medically recognized as they are helping in the treatment of sports injuries, head injuries, chronic pain of the spine and osteoporosis.

Chapter 9

Nutrition

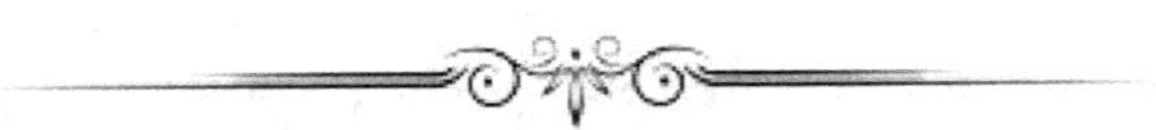

Nutrition is the common name for an entire science, whose roots are dating back to the Latin word - *nutrire* - meaning "to nurture".

In a broader sense it implies consumption of inorganic and organic substances for the purpose of feeding all living beings. With these nutrients, organisms in nature are able to build, renovate and maintain their energy needs. It is one of the conditions where the organisms are kept alive in biological and physiological terms.

Nutrients can generally be in different forms: solid, liquid, semi-solid and gaseous form.

Diet is closely related to many other branches of biology and medicine, such as anatomy (structure of organs), physiology (intake, digestion and metabolism of nutrients and excrementation), evolution (development and adaptation of the system and digestion of nutrients), pathophysiology (which follows the impaired function of the organism as a cause or a consequence of some diseases or intake of food, and diseases caused by it), and sociological component in the nutrition of the human being- (influence of cultural, demographic and religious factors).

The influence of food consumption on a man is very important and crucial to the overall human system, the preservation of health, integrity, social, intellectual and mental abilities.

Every day we become aware of the desperation of those people who are looking for a formula for a proper diet. Everything that does not poison us by consuming it is poisoning us when we try to get rid of it.

The science about nutrition in general is called **dietetics.** The goal of every human being should be to become vegetarian.

Vegetarianism

Vegetarianism is one of the most widespread diets in which people abstain from eating any kind of meat and meat products. Sometimes a person can be radical in vegetarianism, so they will not consume any intermediate products of meat industries such as, for example, gelatin. Their description of what they do not consume can be amazingly simple: do not eat anything that has eyes. But like many other things, so it is about vegetarianism. It is simple only at first glance, because it is significantly more than this simple rule of nutrition. It is a philosophy of life and luxury.

Vegetarianism is described in ancient Greek history from ancient times leading back to the Roman writer Ovid. He incorporated his life philosophy into his historical work "The Metamorphosis". In it, quoting Pythagoras, Ovid says that the condition of progress of humanism lies in the change - in a metamorphosis, which should transform the individuals in that they can sustain a progress in their humanity. Vegetarianism is according to "The Metamorphosis" one of the key decisions, because the lives of humans and animals are so connected, that there is actually no difference between murdering of human beings and animals.

(Ovid: Metamorphoses, Book XV, translated by AD Meeville, Oxford University Press, 1986).

People are usually converting to vegetarianism for very different reasons. Some are due to moral reasons and love or respect for animals, while others encourage health, cultural, aesthetic or religious reasons.

Several variations of vegetarianism are also based upon those reasons, which can be Ovo-vegetarianism (diet includes eggs but not dairy products), Lacto-vegetarianism (which includes dairy products but not eggs), Lacto-Ovo-vegetarianism (which includes the consumption of eggs, milk, milk products and honey), Pescetarianism (including fish consumption and other seafood), Pollotarianism (implies the consumption of poultry meat and other poultry), Pollo-Fish-tarianism (includes consumption of fish and poultry, i.e. "white meat").

The macrobiotic diet is also one type of vegetarianism because it involves mostly full consumption of cereals and legumes. But it can include fish as well. The principle of the diet is also in pursuit of balance or equilibrium between "positive food" (Yin) and "negative food" (Yang).

Essentially the macrobiotic diet is purely vegetarian, because it describes the consumption of meat as "Yang", which could balance if consumed together with sugar which is "Yin". But I think it's a pretty strange and unusual combination, which is not hitting everyone's taste.

These variations of vegetarianism are considered to be semi-vegetarianism.

Veganism

Veganism excludes not only all meat and meat products, but also all food of animal origin. This includes milk and dairy products, i.e., eggs and honey, and also products that have even a trace of animal origin during production such as white refined sugar or products with gelatin.

A very rigorous part of Veganism is known as the Veganism raw diet in which food is permitted only raw and uncooked, meaning unprocessed foods. It includes uncooked fruits, vegetables, seeds and nuts. If certain vegetables are cooked, then cooking is allowed only up to a certain temperature.

Fruitarianism involves consuming only fruits, nuts and seeds provided from plants or trees, but only if done in a manner without damaging the plant or tree.

Vegetarianism in general benefits the health and has wide-ranging benefits for the person that commits to it. This has been documented by the latest scientific work about vegetarianism published 30th January 2013 in the magazine of American Society for Nutrition. It is also the most comprehensive study of its kind, because it covers the study of vegetarians and non-vegetarians during a period of 20 years. The study shows that people who are eating a vegetarian diet are having over 30% fewer diseases of the heart and vascular system.

(F.Crowe, P.Appelby, R.Trevis, F.Key: Risk of hospitalization or death from ischemic heart disease among British vegetarians and non-vegetarians.) 2013

It is also observed that vegetarians have a lower BMI (Body Mass Index), lower blood pressure, and fewer diseases of type 2 diabetes, metabolic syndromes and diseases of the kidney.

It has been shown that consumption of red meat products and processed meat consisting of saturated fat favors the development of esophageal cancer, liver cancer, intestinal cancer and lung cancer.

(A Prospective Study of Red and Processed Meat Intake in Relation to Cancer Risk, PLoS Medicine, 21.04.2008)

Pros and Cons About Vegetarianism and Traps of Vegetarianism

Besides the already described advantages of Vegetarianism, it also reduces the possibility of transmission for many diseases, which are usually transmitted from animals to humans by omnivores, i.e. people whose diet includes meat.

One of the most common and dangerous infections is the one caused by Salmonella. It is estimated that as many as one-third to one-half of the total poultry meat on the U.S. market is infected with Salmonella. Thus, the work of being in the meat industry and the processing of poultry has become one of the most risky

activities in the meat industry.
(JLHill: The Case for Vegetarianism, April 2009)

The second place on the list of a specific infection is beef, which is statistically said to be infected by over 20% with certain forms of cancer that are commonly known under one name as BLV (bovine leukemia virus). The above-mentioned study showed that the BLV and HTLV-1 are the first human retroviruses associated with the development of cancer. Scientific studies have also shown that BIV (Bovine immunodeficiency virus), which is actually a form of AIDS virus in cows, can and is able to infect human cells.

It includes a number of different viruses that can be transmitted by someone eating meat, because processing or proper cooking of the meat cannot eliminate them.

Facts about the danger of infecting humans with distinct viruses that are causing cancer have been growing on importance and are extensively researched around the world.

Vegetarians have a lower intake of B-vitamins with food, so they can have a deficit of vitamin B12, omega-3 fatty acids or EFAs.

Generally the needs of B-vitamins can be covered from

plant sources. By a deficiency of vitamin B12, it must be taken as a substitute because there are no significant B12 sources in food, except in seaweed.

The recommended doses of vitamin B12 are 0.4 mcg (for infants) and 2.8 mcg (for adults). In case of a lack of vitamin B12, which has persisted over a long period and happens to many vegetarians, particularly to vegans, may be a cause for bone weakening.

Eight essential fatty acids which are required for the proper functioning of the body, and that the body cannot produce itself, which means that those must be consumed, can be sufficiently covered through the consumption of Amaranth, Chia-seeds, buckwheat, quinoa, brown rice and hummus.

People that implement a vegan diet can, however, have a lack of some of the amino acids such as a deficiency of DHA (docosahaxenoic acid), which is contained in seaweed. Kelp or seaweed, however, is not suitable for constant consumption due to the high content of iodine. There are some substitutes on the market for that amino acid. Certain types of algae, like spirulina, are good sources of amino acids.

Vegetarians do not necessarily have to be skinny, because they do not consume meat and meat products. Even more, they have to be careful not to feed themselves incorrectly. They should be careful not to consume cheese, whole milk, deep-fried potatoes (French fries), ice creams and chips. Those are all sources of saturated acids, which are harmful to the body.

These are the real hidden traps or Junk food in a vegetarian diet.

Chapter 10

Dietetics

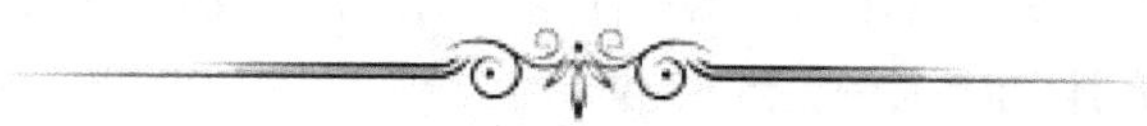

The word dietetics pulls its roots from the Greek language and comes from the word *diaita*, which means "a way of life". The concept has emerged as a common term for all those measures, which encourage a healthful diet for a healthy body.

Today, of course, the notion of dietetics has diametrically changed in its purpose. The present definition of dietetics would incorporate counseling of the patients in terms of a diet counseling that would lead to healing or to represent therapy against certain diseases.

Are you aware of the drama and one of the tragedies of our time?

Thousands of different diets have been written, and the people just "swallow" them because they need better nutrition. People are aware more and more nowadays of the dangers that hang about them in dieting, so they are frenetically searching to find a reliable and healthy diet, which will allow them to maintain their body in a

proper way and have a will to be fed to their satisfaction.
Very few people know what a proper diet contains. Many people even believe they know what a proper diet is, when in fact they do not.

Some people are aware that they do not know what a proper diet is, seeing the evidence of an improper diet on themselves. Both groups of people are rambling from one diet to the other. They are counting calories, drowning themselves with water on a daily basis, not eating any carbs, filling their body with hidden fats by eating processed pre-packed "dietetic" dishes that have little or no carbohydrates. By following diets, such as those that are created and configured to assist the needs of people with diabetes i.e. considering the Glycemic index (GI), or consuming the wrong fats and proteins no matter how carefully the calories are counted, you are bringing your life into jeopardy.

Those who know how to properly nurture themselves are desolately surprised when they see that a proper diet is not completely achieving results. If the information surges in nanoseconds through our thoughts, then it is being transmitted to other cells and it disrupts the flow of bio-energy in the body and the disease occurs in one part of the body that is, by this particular person, a "weak point". Vegetarians, people who are not eating meat, also suffer from cancer or stroke. Because negative emotions like stress of any kind, fear, anger, or trauma, create toxins in the body so that it weakens the immune system, and it cannot overcome the disease.

It is not my intention here to go into the history of dietetics, which would blast the frames of this book, but it is important to note that even Hippocrates of Kos (Greek: Ἱπποκράτης; Hippokrátēs; c. 460 BC) wrote recommendations for various types of diets and therapies, and as he called it "appropriate handling of food and drink."

From his time to today, dietetics has gone through many changes and the influence of the Church, theologians, philosophers and Scholars.

Today is undoubtedly known that food and drink should be in balance with the physical, mental and social needs and abilities of a man.

Natural substitutes and dietary supplements

The human body is supplied with ingredients such as vitamins, minerals and essential amino acids and enzymes. Those are getting into the body through food. The body is synthesizing some of those ingredients itself. Without these ingredients, the body cannot function properly.

Certainly nutrition, environment and age are affecting and having an impact on the supply of the necessary ingredients for the body. Those ingredients are breaking down food and are functioning in very harmonious and most perfect biochemical processes in the biochemical laboratory of our body. There they are fulfilling all the needs of human beings so that the bodily processes are functioning flawlessly.

As long as everything works, we tend not to even notice it and are barely aware of it. When something gets stuck and goes wrong, then it immediately comes to our attention and we remark about the difference between "before" and "now" and all other desires suddenly disappear. An Indian proverb says: "When a person is healthy he has a thousand wishes, when he is ill, he only has one."

If an individual has the comfort and pleasure of being a systemically healthy person, this means there are no serious diseases, and he must try to balance his body and maintain it, in order to stay healthy.

After the age of 50, the body is not active enough to produce certain substances that are necessary for the smooth functioning of the body processes. However, what is most important, the body cannot even infuse from food enough of these substances. Therefore there is a lack of vitamins or minerals as well as essential amino acids and Enzymes in the human body. Depending on where the deficit is, there occurs either minor or long term and major disruptions in the functioning of the human body.

Now, here is information that can save your life: only by taking enzymes on daily basis, you are enabling the resorption of vitamins that you gain either with food or as a supplement. Further, by taking enzymes you are lowering the danger of getting cancer significantly.

However, by the overflow of sales offers for enzymes, which are now readily obtainable on the market, it is hard to make a decision on what to buy. In addition, in Europe it is not possible to obtain some supplies like Enzymes, so people are pretty much left alone. There are doctors, chiropractors, kinesiologists, etc. who have the knowledge and willingness to help people, especially where conventional medicine is not able to. However, there are still not enough of them. On the positive side, holistic medicine, which combines all the knowledge of medical science and deals with the entire human being i.e. analysis of physical, nutritional, environmental, emotional, social, spiritual and lifestyle values, is on the rise.

When you make a decision which product is appropriate for you, you should be sure to have all the facts. As is the case with prescription drugs that are prescribed and applied in conventional medicine, natural dietary supplements may have side effects, which will vary from person to person. It can show itself in a form of skin irritations, headaches, nausea, fatigue, irritability or sensitivity to light.

More to the point, the body of a person consuming natural diet supplements, regardless of which group of supplements, must be able to accept and reprocess the enzymes, vitamins or minerals. And that means that these chemicals should not be consumed at random and in uncontrolled quantities or combinations.

A good example of this is some supplements that include "10 minerals and 10 vitamins." Many people decide to take this supplement because they believe that they have supplied themselves with the necessary daily requirements and don't need to think about that any more. So the manufacturers advertise in their offers that their product in the form of only one pill has it all. However, the human body is not able to synthesize, meaning to rework and store, all these minerals and vitamins that are contained in a single pill. If a person does not have any side effect on a certain supplement, which is anyway rarely the case, it does not mean that the supplement was effective.

Pregnant women and young children should not take

any supplements for a very simple reason: the normal varied diet is sufficient for both groups to synthesize the necessary ingredients from their nutrition. When a person who is pregnant is not consuming any pills unless recommended by their gynecologist, then they will have a better chance for a happy outcome of their pregnancy.

Furthermore, your doctor or pharmacist should review any drug to be sure that the supplements do not react negatively with the prescribed drugs the person is taking. For example, drugs that are taken to lower the concentration of cholesterol - statins, as well as drugs that are taken for lowering blood sugar, are reducing the absorption of the supplement Q10 about which you can read below. If you are taking medications that thin the blood i.e. it does not allow the blood to clot quickly - Cumarin, Coumadin, Warfarin, you should know that at the same time consuming Q10 would reduce the effect of these drugs.

The global market is offering very different natural dietary supplements. The offer is so huge that it is confusing. It offers all sorts of things, so the question is how to choose the right supplement you need that will be effective.

First you need to consider the weakest part of your body, the one that needs support. Then you need to consider your age. As I mentioned, after age of 50, the body does not produce the enzyme that would be sufficient for normal digestion. Or we are producing enough enzymes but our receptors are not functioning. Therefore, you should think about, what is most comfortable for you.

After the age of 50 it is highly recommendable to add Enzymes in a form of supplements to your daily diet.

The following pages should provide you with that help.

When you decide for a particular group of supplements in order to support your body and its functions, then comes the question of what to choose in this ocean of products. Orientation towards products that are already on the market for a longer time should be a good point to start with, because their effects are known and the production is standardized. The effect of the same substances in supplements can vary from different manufacturers. If you prefer one product to another stay with it, and if you start taking a substitute, then take a break for week or two. You should not change to the same product of some other manufacturer because productions are not standardized.

Researches of natural dietary supplements and their functions in the body, have been made, but not under the same standards as medical drugs. Their studies have focused on the main issue - whether or not and how the body can absorb it. The researchers study the ability to accept and recycle particular supplements in the digestive tract of humans and whether these forms of supplements are stable when they reach the digestive tract. If, for example stomach acidity by a particular individual is too high, an enzyme that is taken orally can be destroyed by this elevated acidity, which means that it will be degraded before it can develop any action. An example for this is the enzyme - lipase. This can be avoided if you give priority to a supplement that has specifically covered enzyme capsules.

It is good to take supplements of natural enzymes already made in a certain combination, because in this way a tight interaction between enzymes has been ensured, i.e. they are co working together in a synergistic way and the components are complementing one another.

Vitamins as natural supplements

Vitamins are known to be a part of nutrition allowing the body to attain proper functioning and balance. If you want to know which foods contains which vitamins there is a rich selection of literature on the market. I believe that this would rise above the capacity of this book.

However, if you want to know what it is so important about vitamins as supplements, and the reasons not to take just any vitamins on a random basis, then it is crucial for you to read the next few pages. That means that we cannot just believe that we are meeting the needs of our vitamin intake through our diet and just go with the flow.

Some vitamins are necessary to take in the form of supplements, and some are better to be taken through diet. A specific role in this decision is on an individual basis and the special needs of a person. This shows everywhere all the time and in all situations, because we are all different. Differences between people in this context can show there are different absorptions of nutrients from food or supplements.

Carefully observe and examine your body and in time you will recognize your needs.

I will mention vitamins that are particularly important and whose unnoticed deficit for a long period of time is causing harmful effects, which are then difficult to correct if overlooked unnoticed.

Vitamin D

Vitamin D is the only vitamin that is synthesized by the human body with sun as a catalyst. It is incorporated in food in limited quantities, such as some types of fish specifically mackerel, sardines and tuna. Often it is fortified in some foods such as eggs, milk and juices, which is labeled on the products title that these foods are fortified with vitamin D.

By far the biggest source of vitamin D is gained through exposure of the skin to sunlight. It has been shown, however, that the absorption of vitamin D is reduced in people over age of 50. The safest way to go is to take vitamin D on a daily basis through supplements after a meal in the evening.

Dosages range from 400 IU to 4,000 IU daily.

A deficiency in vitamin D that is not identified for a longer time will result in bone porosity. It is most dangerous for women because with the feminine hormone deficiency at menopause, it leads to osteoporosis.

However, people with certain autoimmune diseases can show a lack of vitamin D. It is known that vitamin D has a positive effect on the function of the immune system and lung function. Historically the treatment with vitamin D has been recognized as a cure against tuberculosis, because it has been found that low or insufficient levels of vitamin D are responsible for development of tuberculosis.

The latest tests have proved influence and correlation between vitamin D and the HIV infection. Also, there are intensive studies in various types of malignant diseases that could be affected by insufficient doses of vitamin D levels.

If you have a viral infection, the oral dose of vitamin D is 800 IU during the first two years, then 2,000 IU of vitamin D daily during the next 12 months.

The clinical science work of the University of Berlin in 2012 has shown that Vitamin D has a positive effect on the treatment of multiple sclerosis.

(J. Dörr, Ohiriaun S., Skarabis H., Paul F., "Eficiacy of Vitamin D supplementation in multiple sclerosis.", 2012)

Besides, vitamin D is acting in the body to regulate some minerals such as phosphorus and calcium.

Also, vitamin D is very significant for persons who have a predilection and weakness for developing Diabetes type 2 and for those who are already having it. Recommended dosage is 400 - 5714 IU daily in the form of a pill, with or without calcium supplements during a period of two months to seven years. A person, however, who already has diabetes, should not take vitamin D without medical supervision.

Levels of vitamin D can be tested in any better equipped laboratory with indicator 25-hydroxyvitamin D. Laboratories in the USA are expressing the value in units of measurement in ng/mL, and other countries are using as units of measurement nmol/L.

A value of 20 ng/mL (50 nmol/L) is considered normal, while those who are above 50 ng/mL (125 nmol/L) should be concerned.

Vitamin C

Vitamin C is ascorbic acid and is one of the essential vitamins in the human body. It is helping the body to absorb iron. The body is not producing it itself, so that intake of vitamin C in form of food or supplements is vital for people. Consumption of one orange or citrus fruit, one large green pepper, or a normal portion of broccoli daily is satisfactory. Everything else is unnecessary and in access: it is excreted in urine because vitamin C cannot be stored in the body.

A normal daily limit intake of vitamin C for adults is between 65 and 90 mg and the top most limit is 2,000 mg / day. In the winter months when the risk of viral infection is higher, it is considered that the intake of 1,000 mg / day should be recommended.

B vitamin

B vitamin includes an entire group of vitamins, so supplements are usually consumed as complexes of B-vitamins. However, I will limit myself to three representatives of the group of B vitamins: Folate (vitamin B9), Vitamin B6 and Vitamin B12

Folate - Vitamin B9

Folic acid, which is a scientific name for vitamin B9, is found in fruits, vegetables, beans, and breakfast cereals. If you take supplements it is recommended that you have a daily intake of 600 micrograms, especially for children, and people whom excessively and constantly enjoy alcohol. This is important because alcohol averts the normal metabolism of folic acid, and as a result this inactivates the folates that should be absorbed in the body. Especially for women, it can lead to breast cancer, as evidenced by recent scientific works in Sweden.

Also the effect of folates in prevention of colon cancer has to be taken into consideration. The latter is still the subject of intense research of scientists around the world. Cancer cells are actually cells of our own bodies that began to uncontrollably flourish and multiply, and studies have shown that these cells need folates for their growth. Therefore, if you have cancer or a precancerous condition carefully decide with your doctor if you should take vitamin supplements.

(Sanjoaquin MA, Allen N, Couto E, Roddam AW, Key TJ: "Folate intake and colorectal cancer risk: a meta-analytical approach", 1997)

Vitamin B6

Intake of this vitamin from the B group of vitamins, which is in medical terms named Pyridoxine, is recommended in a daily dosage between 1.3 and 1.7 milligrams. Very large dosages should be avoided as they lead to nerve damage. The upper dosage limit is 100 mg per day. Such a dose can only be consumed through supplements. But all vitamins of group B are achieving their optimal effect and are best taken through food intake, because B vitamins are generally not absorbed optimally by supplements. Food sources of vitamin B6 are beans, fish, chicken, green vegetables, papaya and orange to name only some of the most important. Vitamin B6 is strongly involved in protein synthesis and is still the object of intensive research in terms of its impact on the reduction of heart diseases.

Vitamin B12

The second name for it is Cobalamin. A daily dosage recommendation should be 2.4 micrograms, and there is no upper limit. It is naturally found in foods of animal origin such as fish, poultry, meat, eggs and dairy products. A deficiency of this vitamin can occur, although almost most people have sufficient or even an excessive intake of this kind of food. The exceptions are vegetarians or vegans, which are a group of people known for a deficiency of vitamin B12. Even if they are taking vitamin B12 as a supplement, some of them are still developing deficiencies, and it happens because some people cannot absorb vitamin B12 in their body. Despite the good quality of B vitamin supplements, you are better off if your source of vitamin B12 is coming through the diet because the absorption of this vitamin is significantly better by nutrition.

Minerals as Natural Supplements

Although there are a large number of minerals known to play a crucial role in human physiology, I will mention the ones that are most important for the balance of the human body.

Calcium

Calcium, together with vitamin D, is a major factor in preventing osteoporosis and generally a part of the normal structure and function of the bones of the human body. Although milk and milk products are considered to be irreplaceable source of calcium, it is not so, which is relieving for those people who cannot or do not want to consume milk and dairy products.

The daily requirement of calcium for adults is 1,000 mg /day, and for women over 50 years of age 1,200 mg /day.

Good sources of calcium are green vegetables, i.e. kale, spinach, broccoli, okra, and almonds and pumpkin seeds. For example: 3/4 cup of kale or spinach has as much calcium as 1 cup of milk.

Zinc

Zinc is known as the mineral that sharpens attention and memory, accelerates wound healing after injury, and also strengthens the immune system. However, one of the most important effects of zinc in the human body is that zinc acts as an antioxidant. Free radicals, which are cruising around the body, are having in their chemical structure one missing electron. So they ramble around the body constantly trying to compensate for one missing electron. They're trying to steal it from the cells and also from DNA. If, or rather when they get successful, this process is called oxidation. Oxidation, which is a normal natural process, is leading to cell aging and to their extinction. Various substances and the mineral zinc are antioxidants, because they prevent the oxidation process, in that they give to the free radicals a missing electron that they are trying to catch, and in this way they actually disable and stop the further oxidation process. Free radicals are no longer seeking to take an electron from cells in the body and thus induce the oxidation process.

In food it can be found in red meat, i.e. beef, lamb, and liver, as well as lobster and oysters. In the group of vegetables and produce, it is to be found in beans, almonds, walnuts, sesame seeds, poppy seeds, celery and mustard.

The recommended dosage of zinc is 50 mg /day. Zinc deficiency is usually caused by lack of food that has it, but can also be caused by the inability to resorb. This is particularly the case by liver and kidney disease, diabetes and some other chronic diseases.

It turned out that some breakfast cereals such as bran cereal containing zinc chelator-phytate are contributing to a lesser absorption of zinc.

(Prasad, AS: "Zinc deficiency", British Medical Journal, 2003)

Magnesium

Consuming the daily requirement of magnesium by individuals is demonstrating itself in an increased memory of the person. However, it should be noted that magnesium is responsible for many very important body processes and is an integral part of the human body: 60% of the magnesium contained is in the bone substance, and 39% is in the cells, correlated with cellular potassium.

The foods that contain magnesium are green vegetables, because they contain chlorophyll. In addition, sources of magnesium are herbs and spices, nuts, coffee, cocoa and tea. Despite the fact that a variety of magnesium products on the market in the form of supplements are huge, overdose is hardly possible because any excess magnesium is immediately excreted from the body through the kidneys. It does not hurt to mention that a well-functioning kidney is essential in supplying the body with ingredients in the form of supplements. A substitute for magnesium is simply taken, as usually it comes, in the form of fizzy tablets.

Normal levels of magnesium in serum are between 0.7 and 1.0 mmol/L, i.e. 1.8-2.4 mEq/L.

It is important to know that both a high and very low protein diet inhibits or prevents the absorption of magnesium in the body.

Results of scientific research, namely meta-analysis, have shown that magnesium deficiency or the inability of the body to synthesize it may be responsible for the more severe forms of depression. In addition, it has been proven that daily intake of magnesium prevents increased blood pressure.

Too low magnesium levels in serum are associated with disease conditions such as metabolic syndrome and type 2 diabetes. A very important role of magnesium is in the reduction of vascular calcification, which is present in people with kidney problems. Magnesium is in fact a natural antagonist of calcium, and magnesium supplementation has been successfully used to prevent the progression of atherosclerosis and is also applied to patients who are on dialysis.

The values of the daily intake of magnesium in the form of natural restitution are between 50 and 150 mg.

Selenium

Simply speaking, selenium is a rare metal, whose salts are toxic in large quantities, but the content of selenium in the body is essential for biochemical processes. Selenium is produced as a byproduct in the production of sulfur and copper in copper refineries and in the process of refining copper. It was discovered in Sweden 1817.

In humans, selenium is a component that is found by humans as a trace element, but it is very important as an antioxidant i.e. that fights against free radicals, as I described previously.

Also, no less important is that selenium participates in the function of the thyroid and allows a proper release of hormones by the thyroid gland in that it releases a rare amino acid called *selenocysteine*.

Selenium may reduce the Hashimoto-syndrome, a disease in which the body attacks the cells of the thyroid gland, as if they were invaders in the body, i.e. an autoimmune disease. Controlled intake of selenium in the form of natural restoration in the amount of 0.2 mg of selenium leads to a reduction of the antibodies that are responsible for Hashimoto-syndrome.

Also important is the molecular mechanism of mercury

poisoning. Recent research has shown that mercury-poisoning causes are irreversible; it means that the inhibition of selenoenzyma whose task is to prevent oxidative damages to the brain and endocrine tissue, are irreversible.

Natural source of selenium are nuts, meat, mushrooms, fish (tuna), shellfish and eggs. It is believed that the level of selenium in the human body is between 13-20 mg.

Coenzyme Q 10

Coenzyme Q10 is a substance similar to vitamins scientifically named Ubiquinone.

Mitochondria are responsible for the transport of the electrons in the cells in form of energy through the human body. 95% of the body's energy is generated by coenzyme Q10. Accordingly, the organs that are the biggest consumers of energy, such as the heart, liver and kidneys, have the highest concentration of coenzyme Q10. Seen from the point of view of science, Q10 was discovered fairly recently. Prof. F. Crane discovered Q10 in 1957 at the University of Wisconsin. It was only four years later, that Peter Michell introduced the true role of CoQ10, for which work he won the Nobel Prize in 1978.

A lack of CoQ10 in the human body appears mainly for two reasons: limited Biosynthesis or increased consumption by the body.

Biosynthesis may be limited due to genetic mutations, mitochondrial mutations, but also by a consumption of statins. This is highly controversial because some drugs are prescribed against elevated cholesterol. CoQ10 follows the same path in the biosynthesis as cholesterol. It is therefore noted that CoQ10 is inhibited in humans that are taking medications such as a beta-blocker and statins. Statins can lower CoQ10 levels in the serum by 40%. Some chronic diseases such as cancer or heart disease are disturbing biosynthesis and are increasing the utilization of CoQ10 in the body. It is currently still the subject of intense scientific research.

Unquestionably it has been proven that taking CoQ10 as a supplement improves heart function and the blood vessel system, reduces high blood pressure, acts as an antioxidant, reduces damage from radiation (shown in experiments), reduces the progress of Parkinson's disease, and prevents migraine attacks, etc.
Daily dose of CoQ10 in the form of a supplement is 50-200 mg.

A natural source of CoQ10 is certainly meat and fish, followed by vegetables as broccoli and cauliflower.

Fruits contain CoQ10 only to some small extent, with the exception of avocado, which has a relatively high content of CoQ10.

In this way the average intake of CoQ10 by natural food has been considered.

The intake through nutrition that comes mainly by eating meat and fish is calculated as 3-6 mg daily.

It is important to note that cooking in oil loses about 30% of CoQ10.

L Glutamine

Glutamine is a nonessential amino acid. In certain health situations it can potentially become essential. This is the case by severe gastrointestinal disorders, such as Crohn's disease, ulcerative colitis and intensive engagement with athletics.

Glutamine has been extensively tested during the last fifteen years. It was found that a part of many important biochemical functions as synthesis of proteins are the source of cellular energy (in addition to glucose), etc.

The biggest consumers of glutamine in human body are

intestinal cells, kidney cells and active cells of the immune system.

Glutamine is used to treat wounds, burns, side effects of tumor diseases, but is also used in all the sports that are based on the increase of muscle mass. In particular, it is recommended in cases of stress, which persist for a longer period of time. It occurs when the body consumes more glutamine than can be produced by muscle. In consequence the same effect can be seen in patients with AIDS.

In order to achieve healing of wounds after traumatic injuries and maintain normal functioning of vital organs, a body needs nitrogen. One-third of the nitrogen comes from glutamine.

Glutamine is in the body stored in the muscle mass, where from there it is transferred into the blood. It is unique, in that it is one of the few amino acids that it is capable of crossing the blood-brain barrier in the brain and cellular barrier in the gut.

It can be found in food in beef, chicken, eggs, milk and dairy products, wheat, cabbage, beans, spinach and parsley.

Glutamine regulates weight by reducing hunger, so that it lowers blood sugar, and helps to burn consumed sugar without being turned into fat.

Omega - 3 fatty acids

Omega-3 fatty acids are essential for normal function of the human body. They belong to the essential fatty acids, which means, the ones that our body cannot produce, so they have to be acquired only by body intake whether it is through food or through supplements.

The foods that contain Omega 3 fatty acids are fish (tuna and salmon, sardines, mackerel, herring), seaweed and olive oil as well as in flaxseed oil, walnuts, walnut oil and pumpkin seed oil.

Consumption of fish is widely known to be beneficial and desirable. Only, it should be consumed in normal quantities, i.e. three times a week. Fish may contain components that are harmful to health, such as mercury and dioxins. It is recommended that only natural fish, i.e. caught in nature and not farmed, be consumed.

The substitution can be taken in the form of fish oil capsules. In this case it is recommended to take capsules containing no more than 3 grams per day of omega-3 fatty acids. Definitely, it is not recommended to take supplements of omega-3 fatty acids without the advice of a doctor, especially if the person has a blood clotting disorder, uses medication to the thin blood (Coumadin) or is taking aspirin. People with diabetes should be taking omega-3 fatty acids in the form of supplements only with the permission of a doctor. The same is true for people who are on medication for lowering cholesterol (Liptor, Mevacor, Zocor).

It is believed that omega-3 fatty acids are helping control all heart diseases and diseases of the blood-vascular system, elevated cholesterol, high blood pressure, diabetes, rheumatoid arthritis, systemic lupus erythematosus, the osteoporosis, depression, bipolar disorder, asthma and inflammatory bowel disease, colon cancer, breast cancer and prostate cancer.

Enzymes

Enzymes are natural catalysts that participate in the biochemical processes in the body, from digestion to DNA synthesis, to name just two of 4,000 biochemical reactions that the enzymes are in control of. In other words, the enzymes are the "fuel" through which all energy reactions in the body take place. In composition terms, the enzymes are mostly proteins, composed of amino acids, which accelerate reactions and energy up to a million times. The list of reactions that are controlled by enzymes would naturally spread the capacity, as well the purpose of this book.

Upon their catalytic activity, enzymes can be divided into two basic groups:

1. Digestive Enzymes
2. Metabolic Enzymes

An important source of enzymes is nutrition. The example for functioning of digestive enzymes is traceable from the moment you put food in your mouth because digestion begins in the mouth. The mouth is the first part of the body, which begins to dissolve the food by digestive enzymes through saliva, which contains the **enzyme Amylase**. This enzyme is starting digestion in that it begins first with the breakdown of carbohydrates. Moving toward the stomach, the proteins from the food that you consumed are broken or split by the enzyme named **Protease**. Milk and dairy products are broken down by the **enzyme Lactase**, which is responsible for the digestion of milk sugar or lactose, which is contained in all dairy foods. The **enzyme Maltase** converts complex sugars from grains into glucose. The **enzyme Sucrase** is continuing degradation of sugars. The **enzyme Lipase** breaks down fats from the food consumed. The **enzyme Cellulase** breaks down fibers. The **enzyme Phytase** generally helps digestion, but especially in a way that is producing B vitamins.

In understanding of the process of digestion, it should be noted that the most common perception by a vast majority of people is that a main part of digestion occurs in the stomach. This impression does not match the facts. Over 90% of the digestive process takes place in duodenum, which connects the stomach with the small intestine. This is actually the beginning of the small intestine.

After consumption of food the stomach gives an indication to the pancreas to excrete digestive juices in the small intestine, i.e. duodenum, to begin the digestion of food. If a person's health is satisfactory or even perfect, the pancreas secretes about 1.5 liters of digestive juices in one day. I am sure you understand why you cannot eat all day long food in large or even in huge quantities. Digestive juices secreted by the pancreas into the small intestine are finally breaking down the food that is already somewhat broken down on the way from the mouth to the stomach.

Those pancreatic enzymes that are secreted by the pancreas into the small intestine could be assorted to three main groups:

Amiolitic Enzyme - breaks down carbs
Proteolytic Enzyme - breaks down proteins
Lipolytic Enzyme - breaks down fat

If the pancreas for any reason (inadequate nourishment, wrong selection and volume of food, age, autoimmune diseases, liver diseases, tumors) is unable to excrete enough digestive juice into the small intestine to break down food, then a passage of food through the gut is too slow. More to the point, the food is not broken down enough, and the growth of bacteria in the small intestine begins. This leads to bloating, fatigue and constipation. It is believed that these conditions are correlated with the disease of Irritable Bowel Syndrome (IBS).

The human body starts decreasing and lowers the production and resorption of enzymes already at an age between 27 and 28. From the age of 50, a person is producing or absorbing only 1/3 of the enzymes amount that one should receive and restore.

To a large extent cooking destroys enzymes. By industrial processing of foods in the process of production due to addition of flavors or additives that should improve the structure, enzymes barely exist. Only foods that contain enzymes are considered bioenergetic food that can bring significant impact on human health.

This is why there are so many supporters of a raw food diet in which people consume food only in its raw form. Personally I do not support anything that radical.

However, it is certain that one particular part of the food you consume daily, must be in its raw form, for example fresh salad.

A normal person, in good physical condition and general health, is recommended to add digestive enzymes to his diet.

If you take digestive enzymes before meals, they will have an impact in the efficient digestion of food. If that same digestive enzyme has been taken between the meals i.e. a few hours after the food consumed and several hours before the next meal, then this enzyme supplement will have an effect through the blood system and work beneficially for the organs.

Metabolic Enzymes are systemic which means that they have a positive effect on organ function, and are manipulating DNA, influencing reproductive cells, cell growth, and affecting those enzymes whose task is only to produce a cellular enzyme.

Enzymes are created by 20 different amino acids, which are specifically arranged. Today, science has been able to clarify the function of DNA and its components, but there are still many open questions.

DNA, or deoxyribonucleic acid through genes, gives a cell a certain model or scheme by which these cells should create enzymes. Created Enzymes are circulating in the cell cytoplasm. If poisons, toxins or tumor cells get involved, the production of Enzymes is blocked.

This can be well explained by the case of antibiotics. An antibiotic is a type of toxic substance whose function is based on the differences between Enzymes in cells of the human body and an Enzyme within a single bacterium. The antibiotic works by destroying bacteria cells, and leaves the cells of the human body intact. Some antibiotics work by destroying the cell wall of bacteria (Penicillin), and some of them in the way that they prevent the enzyme in bacteria to produce nucleotides (sulfonamides). Without nucleotides bacteria cannot multiply.

Enzymes in the battle against cancer

Enzymes that are part of fruit Papaya were used in ancient history in the treatment of tumor growth. Ancient Mayas found evidence of this. Similar traces were also found among Incas and Aztecs.

To understand what connection enzymes are having with tumor cells, we should first make clear that the tumor cells are everywhere in our body, up to 10,000 a day. Rotating, cruising around and looking for a place where they can freely disseminate. It is just that the immune system is not allowing it. Tumor cells differentially diverge from normal cells and are not under the control of other parts of the human body.

The problem comes when a person falls in emotional stress, exposure to pollution of the environment, has poor eating habits, or has been exposed to radiation, etc., because this is the moment when the immune defense system will crash. Tumor cells are of different origins, and this weakens the immune system because it cannot simultaneously defend against so many attackers. It is a moment in which the tumor cells have the opportunity to attach to the cell wall of the normal cell of the body, without immune system being able to detect it.

Tumor cells are very aggressive and self-sufficient. To protect it, tumor cells immediately begin with the formation of a fibrin layer, which is up to 15 times thicker than the layer of normal body cells.

Only enzymes are able to destroy the structure of the fibrin layer, which has the same biochemical structure of fibrin protein as the one piling in the vessels that lead to blockages. A person's immune system is still fighting persistently to create antibodies to new antigens and thus leading to an accumulation of immune complex in the tissues.

Those complexes weaken the immune system entities. Tissue-bound immune Complexes are found in people with autoimmune diseases, tumors and infections.

Application of the Enzymes under normal and proper nutrition allows tissue-bound immune complexes to set themselves free from tissue and enable macrophages to release TNF - tumor necrotic factor that destroys fibrin cover of tumor cells.

Chapter 11

When, How, Why and What To Eat

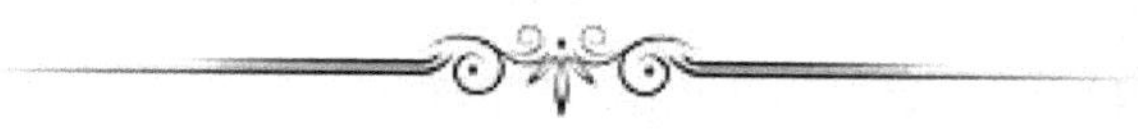

There is no standardized formula for what or when to eat, as human nutrition is an individual thing. It is ruled by your own taste and some people who suffer from certain diseases such as diabetes yet can determine options also. And as a consequence this might determine and establish a person's way of supplying and nurturing himself. An individual metabolic type is also having a crucial role that would decide a person's diet. The metabolic type of a person will depend on what kind of diet would be ideal for that type of person. This is one of the main reasons why diverse diets cannot be successful: not everything is for everyone.

I will talk about **when you do not need to eat**, and **what are the main metabolic types of people.**

Commonly all advice about dieting start with common rules on nutrition in terms that they are talking about the food that should be consumed in order to attain a balanced diet, and thus be optimum for the body. All possible diets are relating mostly about what to eat.

I will first start with what not to eat, and when you should not eat because I think it is much more important.

In the first place it is necessary to know how organs, that are vital for digestion in your body, are functioning. You should have tests conducted to ensure your organs are healthy. Only when you are convinced that your test values of the vital organs are normal can you conclude, if you have no other subjective difficulties, that your organs are functioning normally.

Metabolism is by definition the chemical processes occurring within a living cell or organism that are necessary for the maintenance of life. In metabolism some substances are broken down to yield energy for vital processes while other substances, necessary for life, are synthesized. Chemical reactions in the body's metabolic processes are obtainable with the help of Enzymes as a medium, which is to be understood as chemical modification and exchange of goods.

If you have checked the value of your vital organs and they are normal, or only slightly deviating from normal, and you still have subjective difficulties in terms of weight gain, difficulties with digestion after consuming food, constipation or diarrhea, then you can suffer from **metabolic syndrome.** This means you might lack of one or more **enzymes, hormonal imbalance**, or you are doing something wrong.

Metabolic Types of People

Although each person is different from another, there are still common traits in a very broad scope of individual distinctiveness that consists of three basic metabolic groups of people.

It is the turning point, where a large percentage of diets offered on the market turn out to be a failure at least for you and me. If you get rid of the weight, you will probably get it back. This happens only because certain foods are eaten, depending on the rules of a specific diet, which does not take into account an individual's metabolic type, and specific requirements, i.e. different needs of each person.

Metabolic types of individuals have been first described in **Ayurveda** and are certainly worth mentioning. Although very extensive, anyone can find himself or herself described in one of three metabolic types, which are called Doshas in Auyrveda.

When you start searching to find which metabolic type of person you are, i.e. to which Dosha, you are beginning the first step toward the direction of proper nutrition. The type of person will not be determined only by the physical characteristics (shape, structure,

metabolism of the body), but also by mental and psychological characteristics.
Doshas are actually defense mechanisms of the body that is in a constant state of balance. In the beginning, you will be confused because you will find in each Dosha something that matches yourself, a part that belongs to you, and then, at the same time many features that are not compatible with your person.

This is because; everyone has all three doshas.

The characteristics of one person are manifesting themselves not only by the type of metabolism and body build, but also by the energy consumption and its balance or imbalance.

Any disease is the result of an imbalance.

Some doshas are characteristic for specific diseases, which a person is experiencing. So if you cannot say with certainty what type of person you are or to which dosha you belong, i.e. in which features and characteristic of this particular dosha you can identify yourself with, you will be able to determine it easily by disease.

It is always one Dosha, which is responsible for a particular disease because of its over-dominant effects. But in the background of the issues, all three doshas are actually always in disproportion.

When the body is in a state of homeostasis (a balanced state of the body, with no change), then we can say that a person is in a state of health.

Doshas are in a state of homeostasis and are silent and invisible. The body is complementing itself in homeostasis, correcting processes and healing itself. If there is a Dosha, which is prevailing, there will be an imbalance and disease occurs.

The three Doshas are Vata, Pitta and Kapha.

Vata Dosha

If 5 or more characteristics of this Dosha apply to you, then this is a type and constitution of the body to which you belong. Of particular significance are features of the body structure.

* Narrow to petite body shape
* Lighter weight and small bone constitution, often thin or malnourished
* Dry and rough skin, darker skin, depending on race
* Brown to black hair color
* Bigger teeth with light enamel, often uneven due to lack of space, possible protrusion of the upper front jaw and/or overbite

* Smaller and thinner lips
* Dark eyes
* Rapid speech and movements
* Developed creativity and imagination
* Slightly sweating
* Poor appetite, changeable and irregular nutrition
* Tendency to constipation and frequent bloating, problems with the function of the bowel
* Susceptible to concerns, fears, and disorders of the nervous system, easy entry into depression and stress
* Very strong sex drive or no sex drive
* Tendency to arthritis
* Love to travel
* Do not like cold water
* Tendency to dehydration

When Vata prevails and is not in balance, there are disorders such as dehydration, arthritis, or disorders of the intestine, because a dehydrated body has a greater need for water. There is not enough water to soften the feces in the intestine and this leads to the formation of gas and constipation. Signs are dry skin, a tendency to lose hair, or white spots on the nails.

Also, an increased or misbalanced functioning of the Vata affects the mind, so that they think very quickly and the person is highly stimulated. Thoughts are swarming in their head, and it is easy to create fear and apprehension because the imagination is enhanced.

This person is prone to develop depression. A Vata person is very quick and easy to understand things and events around themselves, and with the same speed they easily forget, because while they are discussing one thing there are ten other things are on their mind.

How and when to feed yourself, if you are a Vata type of person?
How to deliberately help the Vata person not to get out of balance?

° It is urgently required to achieve order and routine in their everyday life, and that means discipline in the schedule of sleeping and eating.

° A day should be started with a glass of lukewarm water with two to three tablespoons of freshly squeezed lemon juice - it cleans the liver

° Never skip breakfast, no matter how minor it is. This means that it may only consist of vegetables processed in a good juicer. Or you can add half a banana to get your drink more condensed. Or you may add honey.

Examine carefully your food intolerance, and the best way to do this is to arrange for the Enzyme-linked Immunosorbent Assay (Elisa) test to determine your intolerance on certain types of food. Check whether it is good for you to consume milk and milk products at all.

Considering cereals, you should be moderate and careful. The Vata-people are not good in digesting some starches (potato) and corn.

You will find recipes in the last chapter.

A selection of recipes will be published in a special book about the BBB diet most likely the end of 2013.

° Vata people need to eat sweets (not necessarily sugar, especially not white sugar). They also should consume sour and salty foods, if the condition of the body allows it.

° They need to stay warm and dressed in comfortable clothes

° They must make sure that their body is hydrated, i.e. to take plenty of fluids daily in small quantities.

° Vata people do not digest raw foods and vegetables such as lettuce well. So they should eat salad chopped into strips in moderate portions.

° Beans, nuts and potatoes should be avoided.

° They should do daily skin care.

° They should not skip meals, do not eat often, but not

even huge portions.

° Vata people should avoid laxatives and bowel cleansers.

The word Vata literally translated means wind. The element of a Vata person is air, so this shows that the Vata Dosha is very unstable and can easily fall out of harmony.

Pitta Dosha

If 5 or more characteristics of this Dosha apply to you, then this is a type and constitution of the body to which you belong. Of particular significance are features of the body structure.

* Medium body build
* Normal bone structure and body
* Average to higher tallness
* Medium weight or increased weight, depending on whether the person possibly has a metabolic problem
* Slightly smaller sized yellowish teeth
* average size of mouth
* Green or gray-ashen eyes
* Very clear articulate voice
* The skin is often lighter and can have freckles, rosy cheeks
* Hair is lighter, brunette and people are often

redheads
* Very intelligent
* Have a brilliant sharp mind
* Ambitious
* Have an excellent memory
* Jealous
* Prone to sweating
* Have a strong appetite
* Very passionate sex
* Feces is of softer consistency / diarrhea
* Often have problems with eyesight and are wearing glasses
* Do not like hot water
* Love luxury
* Does not like a mess, they are always cleaning all around

A Pitta person is mainly preoccupied with everything that is related to digestion. This means that they also create stomach acid or bile very emphatically. When Pitta prevails and is not in balance, it leads to digestion disorders such as reflux, stomach ulcers or gallstones. These disorders are happening when the digestion is in an imbalance in terms of being slow. As a result, food stays longer in the small intestine than it would otherwise, and this increases the number of bacteria. Acidity is the result. To overcome this situation, the body introduces a self-correction and enhances the work of Pitta Dosha.

However, this is not the end. As a result of an increased activity of the Pitta Dosha due to lazy digestion and accumulation of bacteria in the small intestine, there is often a leakage of the intestinal wall and bacteria enters the bloodstream. This opens the way to all kinds of inflammations in the body, which can take various forms and locations. Propensity to inflammation in the body is a very dangerous situation if repeated, even if it is of low intensity, so that the person is not aware that the inflammation. As a result, the person becomes very irritable, and shows diseases of the skin, such as redness of the skin, hives and eczema. It can lead to the outbreak of psoriasis, which is also linked to shocking and stressful events.

High blood pressure and headaches or migraines, and redness around the eyes are possible also.

In the mental component the person can appear as being very hyper, very critical toward their environment, fighting for positions, rivalry, workaholic, insisting on their own rules and own principles and are displaying intolerant behavior. When in imbalance, a Pitta person can often be unbearable for others in their environment. They are very omnipresent, conscious and awake. One would say they are not wasting any opportunity to act or react.

Their digestion and the internal secretions of the body, which is the main feature of Pitta people, intensifies around noon and midnight developing in a range of two hours before and after. Therefore, the Pitta person is very active and known as "night owls" because they work, learn, read or burn the midnight oil.

This activity by Pitta Dosha is meant to be used at this time of night by the body for digestion and for cleansing of the organs (e.g. liver). So the Pitta person is actually "stealing" the energy of his own body. This may work well for a long time until the person is brought to stress or illness that weakens the immune system.

With its system of self-regulation, Pitta Dosha is trying to regulate it in a way that enhances its activity. In this case there is a disbalance and a person has the disease. The vulnerability of Pitta people is their digestive organs - mainly the stomach and liver. On the second place is undoubtedly a risk of inflammation in the body. If inflammation persists or is repeated, it comes to the development of cancer, which has been scientifically proven.

Intensified work by the Pitta Dosha about 10 o'clock at night leads to acidifying of the body due to increased secretion of gastric acid and bile. This leads to discomfort and the Pitta person likes very much to eat some dessert or something sweet two hours after dinner. Sweets are minimizing their feeling of discomfort.

This can have a negative impact on the person's weight. Pitta persons may have excess weight, which can be seen throughout the body if they are a pituitary type of person. Or there is a very pronounced increase in weight in the hips and thighs if they are a gonadotropic type of person. If a person shows signs of weight gain, which are particularly indicated in the waist, then it is a metabolic syndrome, which will be specifically described in the following sections. It is one of the most important sets of factors that are responsible for the development of obesity because people cannot process food properly. This inevitably leads to the emergence of type 2 diabetes, which if is not stopped creates the vicious circle leading to type 1 diabetes. Further, as a result of this vicious circle, it leads to disturbances of the liver values, elevated blood fats, high blood pressure, heart attack or stroke.

If you are in an awkward situation, because you know that this is your problem, do not despair, but make yourself committed to controlling your life. In your everyday life it means that you need a plan. If you have a plan, then your mind is busy with the organization to realize this plan, so you do not have time to think about it, or to be unhappy. There are a lot worse things than that. And this you may know yourselves.

Pitta people are well-organized, conscious and responsible persons. These characteristics are not so prominent in their youth, but are showing significant progress with growing up and aging.

How and when to feed yourself if you are a Pitta type of person?
How to consciously help the Pitta person not to get out of balance?
° For breakfast they must eat something of stiffer consistency, such as a banana or grated apple and a cup of coffee or tea. Or, you can eat a piece of dark homemade baked bread, if you eat bread and cereals. Liquids must be consumed more often, specifically in the summer months when the temperatures are higher, otherwise only when necessary. It is up to your choice.

° Daily meals can be arranged according to your daily time table, but be sure to be finished with dinner by eight o'clock in the evening. Beyond that time, simply lock the kitchen. No deserts around 10pm.

° Avoid various oils except olive oil. Do not use it in baking because in that form olive oil harms the body. If you love to eat food from a Wok, pour a little water into the wok after heating it well and then insert the vegetables. Then a few minutes after you sauté the vegetables in boiling hot water, which will soon evaporate, add the virgin olive oil.

Other oils are to be avoided, because they reinforce negative effects if the Pitta is out of balance, except pure organic coconut oil. You can consume as well a limited amount of fresh organic butter or even better - ghee.

° Cheese, tomatoes, chili peppers, cucumbers and peanuts are not forbidden by Pitta people, but it is good to avoid them, or at least eat those very rarely. If you are not "Fit", try not to eat the foods mentioned.

° Do not drink alcohol or at least reduce it to a minimum

° Avoid black coffee, or at least reduce it

° Do not consume vinegar or a mixture of vinegar

° Do not eat food that is too hot

° salt your food moderately, or avoid it altogether

° intentionally eat bitter foods, or as often as you can: nonalcoholic aperitifs, Cynar, salad radicchio, cooked chicory and fresh steamed artichokes.

° Regularly go to bed at about 10 o'clock in the evening

Kapha Dosha

If 5 or more characteristics of this Dosha apply to you, then this is a type and constitution of the body to which you belong. Of particular significance are the features of the body structure.

* Sturdy physique constitution
* Heavy bones and well-built skeleton
* People can appear as huge, due to large skeleton
* Mostly overweight, leaning to be overweight
* Very strong and healthy
* Has bad breath
* Full lips and big mouth
* Usually have blue eyes
* Have a quiet, monotonous and rather boring voice, speaks slowly
* Have thickened pale and oily skin
* Have increased sweating
* Have a good memory
* Have a need for a deep and long sleep
* Generally are sleeping too long
* Are loyal and reliable
* Stools are heavy and soft
* Have a good appetite
* Usually successful as businessmen / women

* Are very passive
* Do not like the cold
* Love good food and delicacies
* Prefer to stay in the family and are a "pillar" of the family

Kapha persons have an increased production of mucous, i.e. slime, everywhere in the body where grease and fat cells normally are. Their digestion is very slow and sluggish, and circulation is very weak. They love to eat and reach for food even when they are not hungry, because it calms them down. They are having a tendency to retain water in the body, and prone to edema and puffiness, and as a consequence can have increased volume of breast tissue.

If they are in imbalance, their symptoms increase, so they may cross over into developing a disease.

Kapha people have an overgrowth of the mucosa wherever mucosa cells are located in the body. So it is starting from the head and sinuses through the entire digestive tract. Thus, they can suffer from frequent sinusitis, which thickens the lining, leading to inflammation of the sinuses, bronchi and the entire respiratory tract. If inflammation of the respiratory tract is not prevented and minimized, and if it lasts a longer time, there is a thickening of the lining inside of the nose and sinuses, which solidify, and in very severe cases leads to chronic inflammation of the respiratory tract, especially of the nose and sinuses. Increased mucus in the mouth enhances the desire for food, and mucus in the stomach makes digestion slow. It all affects breathing, as the lungs and the entire digestive tract are full of excessive mucus.

They often have a decreased function of the thyroid gland and thyroid hormones; which is further increasing the risk of obesity.

Water retention in the body is weakening the functioning of all organs, and hyperglycemia occurs. The pancreas has to work more intensively and eventually this leads to diabetes type 2, which then turns into diabetes type 1, because the pancreas cells completely cease to secrete insulin.

Kapha people are also having an increased concentration of cholesterol in the blood so that the blood is getting thicker. They are prone to have blood clots in their vessels or a vessel diameter is narrowing, and consequently the poor circulation becomes even weaker. Their feet are always cold, which is of course due to poor circulation.

The density of blood has an effect on the mind and mood. Persons under the influence of a stronger Kapha Dosha can have grim thoughts, which if persisting can cause depression. People instinctively grab desserts, cakes, chocolate or ice cream, because it then calms them down somewhat and makes them satisfied.

How and when to feed yourself if you are Kapha-type of person? How to deliberately help Kapha not to get out of balance?

° Kapha people should start their day by getting up early, in order to comply with the functioning of their body with circadian rhythm. Also, for them the best thing to do after getting up is to immediately go to the gym or take part in some physical activity of their choice. At least fifteen minutes, or half an hour is ideal.

°They should eat completely unsalted food or at least reduce the consumption of salt to the minimum

° For the Kapha person a vegetarian diet is optimal. If it is not acceptable, then they should avoid the consumption of meat and meat products after 5 o'clock in the afternoon.

° It is also preferable to avoid milk and dairy products. If this is not acceptable, those products should not be consumed after 5 pm.

° They need to reduce the consumption of wheat products after 5 pm. This of course implies not only to bread, but also all food containing dough.

° They should avoid foods with sugar, sweets, cakes, creams, ice cream, etc. Also be aware of sugars, which are hidden in instant drinks such as coffee or cocoa, as they contain glucose as a sweetener.

Especially dangerous are coffee drinks containing whipped cream on top. It has become very modern, in recent years, to see people, mostly young and middle-aged, with disposable cups, drinking these beverages along the way. And the calories that we consume "on the run" are never counted or taken into consideration of the daily calorie intake, even if you ask that person what they have consumed during day. One such cup with cream and add-ons contain 300 to 1200 kcal. This makes the liver work hard, and because of poor absorption the excess sugar turns into fat cells.

° They should be avoiding or completely stop eating all kinds of sweetened drinks, juices, sodas, and artificially sweetened juices. As a sweetener, it is best to use Stevia.

The so-called liquid sugars, especially fructose, are dangerous for the organs that are processing sugars (liver and pancreas). Natural fruit juices such as fresh orange juice, should be consumed very controlled or not at all. The exception is natural lemon juice. Lemon is the only citrus fruit that creates alkali conditions in the body.

° They should completely avoid all foods prepared in deep oil that are served as a deep-fried food.

° Kapha people should consume lean prepared meals and pay attention to the use of oil. It is very beneficial if you limit yourself to consume organic olive oil, which is provided under the label "extra virgin olive oil "(which means that this olive oil is pressed from olives without the use of heat or chemicals). Such olive oil is beneficial when used properly, because it is decreasing the levels of cholesterol in the blood and has a positive effect on the heart, protection of the liver and the immune system.

° They should avoid acidic foods and the use of vinegar. Many top cooks can very deliciously season everything with squeezed lemon juice, which is not really an alternative choice, but used in the preparations of most delicious delicacies.

° They should consume freshly squeezed lemon juice daily, starting their morning with a teaspoon of lemon juice with luke water on an empty stomach, using it as dressing for salads and marinades, and regularly putting a few drops in a clear vegetable, chicken or beef soup. Lemon juice should be consumed each day.

This allows the creation of alkali conditions in the body and is cleansing your liver, which is especially by Kapha person a weak point, as are all the vital organs in the body.

However, as I mentioned earlier, everyone has the elements of all three types of Doshas. The only question is which elements will prevail under consideration of a person's constitution.

Since lemon juice not only works by preventing acid in the body and cleanses one of our most important organs - the liver daily, it is also proven to have 20 anticancer components. Therefore it should be regularly included in a diet of all people in a way that I have described.

To understand Metabolic Syndrome, we must first explain the role of the hormone, Cortisol, in the body.

The Effect of Cortisol

Cortisol is a hormone, a product in the human body in the cortex of adrenal gland. It is synthesized actually from cholesterol, and named after the crust of the adrenal gland - Cortex. Popularly referred to as the "stress hormone", it works in correlation with other hormones and amino acids, and is responsible for the breakdown of glycogen to glucose in the liver and muscles. One of its many functions is to reduce inflammation in the body. Because of its effectiveness against inflammation it is often applied in wide use and unfortunately without a prescription as a remedy for helping with some skin problems (such as eczema) and arthritis.

However, as I previously mentioned, cortisol is released from the adrenal gland cortex as a response to stress. This happens because being in stress the body is endangered, and cortisol is having a suppressing function to insulin, which is breaking down sugar in the blood. This leads to hyperglycemia, i.e. an increase of sugar levels in the blood. As a result, processing of sugar starts to develop in the liver. This is leading to so-called insulin resistance. It is a condition in which insulin cannot perform its function, which is to carry the sugar into the cells in order to supply them with the food, i.e. energy. The cells are unable to take glucose, amino acids and fatty acids, so that they can "cure" the cells. The cause for this is the reduced number of glucose transporters in the cell membrane called GLUT-4. Cortisol is using this mechanism as a response to stress in order to protect the body, considering that the body is under stress. This means that the body is having an emergency situation so that residual glucose is needed for brain function.

However one of the most devastating results and consequences of cortisol is the damaging impact on the immune system, simply because the functioning of the immune system, in an emergency situation, where the body is fighting to survive, is not a priority anymore. This entails an enormous number of important processes in the body. If the organism is exposed to cortisol for a long time, then it comes up with conditions and diseases that are life threatening.

The problem is also that the hormone cortisol has a joint reaction with adrenaline. It creates a memory of recently experienced emotional events of the person that is stored in the cells. It serves the memory in order to know what to avoid in the future. But if such information's are stored for a longer period of time, they are damaging a part of the brain where they are stored, called the hippocampus. In this part of the brain is the learning center.

In further action Cortisol increases blood pressure and

affects the increase of appetite and obesity.

The values of cortisol levels around 9 am are between 140 nmol / L, which is the lowest lower limit and 700 nmol / L. which is the highest upper limit. At midnight, the lowest lower limit of cortisol is 80 nmol / L and the highest upper limit is 350 nmol / L.

What can you do if the cortisol level is too high? The supplement magnesium taken after aerobic exercise lowers cortisol. Also, massage therapy, music therapy, regular dancing, humor and laughter can also lower cortisol.

Factors affecting the increase in cortisol levels are not enough sleep, too intense physical exercise, postmenopausal hormonal therapy, stress that lasts a long time and is repeated over a long period of time, severe trauma and a significant reduction in caloric intake.

Scientific work in 2010 has proven that the level of cortisol in serum, i.e. in the blood, can predict mortality from cardiovascular accident or stroke.

Metabolic syndrome

Metabolic syndrome is also known under the names

Insulin Resistance Syndrome or Syndrome X. It is a combination of medical unbalanced conditions, which if they occur in this combination, are having an incredibly dangerous effect on the development of cardiovascular disease or stroke. The syndrome is so dangerous, and so widespread (Estimated to be spread to more than 25% of all residents in the USA, and over the age of 50 years as much as 44% of the population suffers from the syndrome), it represents a major threat to human health. Individuals that are suffering from Metabolic Syndrome have been scientifically proven to have a certain genetic code. It is, however, makeable to interrupt this vicious cycle of symptoms in that person acquires a certain way of dieting, i.e. sustenance. In this way, one can prevent the further development of the disease in the chain of Metabolic Syndrome.

Not only are these statistical figures frightening, moreover the majority of associated causes of this syndrome have been put together only recently, which is terrifying.

You can say with almost certainty that you are suffering from Metabolic Syndrome if you have three or more of the following symptoms:

* Waist circumference greater than 102 cm (40 inches) in men and waist circumference greater than 88 cm (35 inches) in women and tendency to gain weight in the

abdomen
* Triglycerides values - equal to or greater than 150 mg / dl (1.7 mmol / L)
* Reduced HDL ("good") cholesterol:
  - Men - less than 40 mh / dL (1.3 mml / L)
  - Women - Less than 50 mg / dL (1.29 mml / L)
* Increased blood pressure: equal to, or greater than 130/85 mm Hg, or being on drugs
* Increased fasting glucose: equal to or greater than 100 mg / dL,
  5.6.mmol / L or being on drugs

If in addition to the described symptoms above you have increased markers for systemic inflammation in the body - CRP - C-Reactive Protein, then it is almost unquestionably that you have to deal with the Metabolic Syndrome.

In addition to that, markers such as Fibrinogen and Interleukin 6 can show increased levels.

Recent scientific works in the field of neurobiology have discovered that the base and one of the causes of metabolic syndrome is stress. No matter what kind of stress it is: whether it is physical or psychosocial, it disrupts the balance of hormones of the HPA-axis.

HPA-axis is the hypothalamic-pituitary-adrenalin axis whose interaction works as follows:

- HPA-axis increased activity is resulting in higher values of cortisol in the blood circulation. This is causing elevation of glucose and insulin, which leads to an accumulation of fat around the organs (Visceral fat - fat accumulation around the organs thereby it is increasing the volume of the waist):
- Further it leads to insulin resistance and high blood pressure. That way the circuit of Metabolic Syndrome is closed, which consequently leads to cardiovascular disease, type 2 diabetes and stroke.

The importance of the proper functioning of the HPA-axis is that it is one of the main parts of the neuroendocrine system, which is not only controlling the stress reactions, but is also regulating many body processes, including digestion, the functioning of the immune system, emotions, etc.

By healthy people, the level of cortisol rises sharply after waking up and after a half hour it is reaching the peak, after which is slowly falling through the day, and rising again later in the evening. This is called Circadian Cycle Rhythm. Late in the evening cortisol value fall again and reach the lowest value in the middle of the night.

Abnormal circulation of the cortisol cycle in the body is associated with illnesses such as Chronic Fatigue Syndrome, Insomnia and Burnout. Also unhealthy functioning of the HPA-axis is closely related to neurobiology and is widely spread in a number of mood disorders and functional disorders such as depression, irritable bowel syndrome, PTSD, etc.

Experiments have shown that fish produce the same cycle of hormones of the HPA-axis, when they are under more stress due to enduring endangerment by another dominant fish. An example is the shading of skin that occurs under stress in some species of salmon: the HPA-axis is deactivating itself to suppress aggression. One of the amino acids that act to suppress aggression and greater resistance to stress is L-tryptophan.

But let's leave the fish alone; let's go back to the people.

The stress hormone cortisol is produced in the adrenal gland. In stress situations, i.e. uncontrolled situations that are compromising the integrity of the person, cortisol is below the normal levels in the morning, and is elevated or above normal levels in the evening.

Circadian Rhythm, or Circadian Biological Clock

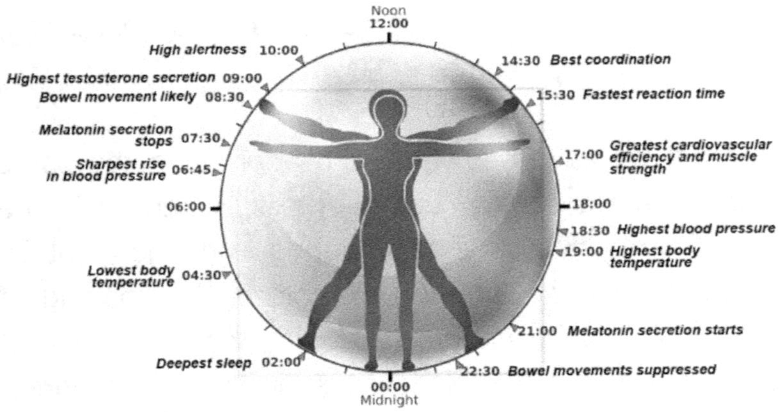

Circadian Rhythm is a kind of biological clock that affects the physiological processes in the body. Those are fluctuations in the body, which are taking place without our will. It is important to know that the circadian rhythm cannot be adjusted, or be modified to a different functioning and different oscillations. Pilots, flight staff and the "jet set" that are changing time zones often suffer from changes in the circadian rhythm, which is known as jet lag.

The Biological clock is affected by several factors, one of which is a day and night switch over, or the influence of light. Besides, the levels of the hormone cortisol in the blood affect the biological clock. The biological clock or Circadian Rhythm is stimulating the sense of hunger, which is centered and run by the gland Hypothalamus. The feeling of hunger may be disrupted if either of the hormones Ghrelin and Leptin is not functioning properly as regulators for the feeling of hunger / satiety. As a result of those two hormones being disturbed, their secretion leads to misinformation. The example for this is when those hormones are not secreted, and the person is not getting the signal of being full and keeps eating.

The Biological clock of each person determines body temperature, appetite, alertness, hormone secretion, excremention, thirst and bedtime.

Moreover, the results show that every cell in the body has its own autonomous biological clock. Cells, as previously mentioned, communicate with each other.

Disorders of the Circadian Rhythm, or Biological clock in humans can lead to a serious metabolic imbalance, which then disturbs many other factors and is difficult to put in order. Or a disorder of the digestive system occurs, because "wrong signals" are being exchanged among the cells. Cells have receptors: those in the eye are receptive to light, which is one aspect of the biological clock, and those in the liver have receptors for food. This information then, which has been exchanged, is deciding about how much you sleep, when you wake up and when you feel hungry.

In conclusion, this fact and the described mechanisms of the biological clock in the human body, a person should not feed themselves at a time when the biological clock is in a standby mode, i.e. at night. Everyone knows the example of some people who feel hungry and eat in the middle of the night. This is an alarming example of circadian rhythm disorder.

It is very damaging that some articles, daily newspapers and other publications publicly and quite illogically advise people that it does not matter what time of the day or night someone eats. Not only is this food consumption harmful to the person, but also the goal should be for every human being to shape and define his or her daily habits, which will then eventually have a positive impact on the Circadian Rhythm. Get used as much as possible to take your meals at approximately the same time each day. You should not eat by any means when you are not hungry or just because it is "time" to eat. You are free to skip a meal if you do not feel hungry. The signal for hunger, as I previously mentioned, arises through secretion of two hormones - *ghrelin* and *leptin*.

Ghrelin is an amino acid and a hormone discovered relatively recently (1997). It is the product of gastric cells and Y cells in the pancreas. If Ghrelin is secreted excessively, it has a negative effect on the signaling of satiety and inhibits the vagal receptors, so these people are gorging themselves i.e. they do not have the feeling that they ate enough and cannot stop eating.

Ghrelin is significant because, in addition of its impact on hunger and the need for increased consumption of food, it is very significantly determining the participation of the pituitary gland in the brain in reference to cognitive adaptation of humans on their environment and the ability to learn. The ability to learn is closely correlated with ghrelin and is best in the morning and during the day when the stomach is empty, because then the concentration of ghrelin is at the highest levels.

However, experiments on laboratory mice have shown that the concentration of ghrelin is significantly elevated in chronic stress. Indeed, elevated ghrelin levels by stress remain high during the next four or more weeks.

Levels of ghrelin increase between midnight and early morning hours in people of normal weight and those who are have a thin body type. However, in obese people, this is indicating the dysfunction and failure in the system of the circadian rhythm. The significantly increased level of ghrelin is caused by the lack of proper sleeping hours, which increases appetite and reduces the production of leptin, which on the other hand suppresses appetite.

Recent research has examined the effects and side

effects of gastric bypass surgery. It has been shown that it does not only reduce the capacity of the stomach, but it also dramatically reduces the levels of ghrelin compared with lean subjects, whether they have naturally skinny constitution, or have lost a weight by weight diet.

In addition, ghrelin plays a major role in the suppression of inflammation, oxidative stress, damage to the lining of the stomach and intestinal inflammation (colitis).

Leptin is a protein consisting of 167 amino acids in humans and is located in chromosome No 7. It was discovered in the USA in 1994. Except for some processes and synthesis in which it participates, leptin is responsible for a decrease in appetite. In very obese people leptin is significantly increased, which is scientifically explaining the resistance to leptin. Similar to insulin resistance, when a person produces insulin, the receptors to receive hormones have failed.

An example of this are the recent studies that have proven that consuming fructose, especially large quantities daily, leads to leptin resistance in experiments, as well as to the increased value of triglycerides. Values were significantly greater in the group of animals that were fed fructose than in the group of animals that have been fed with fat and high-calorie foods. Therefore, I must emphasize: fruits in limited quantities, yes, but certainly not 3 to 5 servings a day!

(Science News. Science Daily: Fructose Sets Table For Weight Gain Without Warning, "2008)
(Shapiro et al. "Fructose-induced leptin resistance exacerbates weight gain in response," 2008)

By healthy people leptin values are between 1 and 5 ng/dl by men, and 7-13 ng/dl by women.

The dynamics of leptin changes significantly by acute changes of bioenergetic balance or equilibrium.

(Int.journal of Obesity, Keim, Stern, Havel, Kok: "Fasting leptin and appetite responses induced by a 4-day 65% of the energy deficit in women", 2006)

Brazilian researchers have proven that melatonin increases leptin levels only in the presence of insulin, and therefore causes a decrease in appetite during sleep. However, the mice with diabetes type 1, who were treated in the experiments either with leptin or with leptin in combination with insulin, showed healing. Obviously it takes a lot of testing, but it seems that a new page in science has been opened and so a hope for the treatment of diabetes.

A Circadian Rhythm is 1 CR, which is equal to 24 hours 11 minutes and 16 seconds. The Circadian Rhythm that biological clock is embedded in the space shuttle, for the astronauts on space flights.

Chapter 12

Bioenergy and food

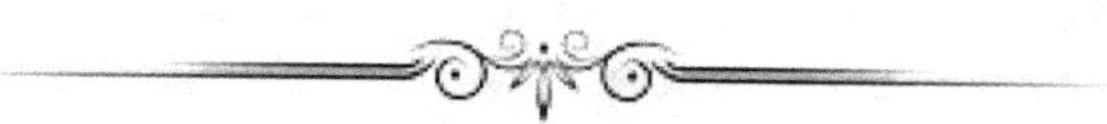

Foods that we consume also contain bioenergy. Or they are supposed to contain it. If we are talking of genetically manipulated products about which so much has been written and spoken and which battles are being fought in the media and in the courts, then we can surely not say this food is bioenergeticly balanced.

When growing food, fruits, grains and crops that are not genetically manipulated, only food and products that carry the label "Bio" or "organic" guarantee bioenergy value.

A good thing to start with is to get a proper selection of foods that are in bioenergetic balance, i.e. that are naturally grown and are not genetically manipulated and treated with chemicals and pesticides which are highly toxic and harmful to human health.

The next step to follow is how to properly prepare these foods.

To summarize what was said previously, the first step is to be focused on your choice of your ingredients, which follows with the correct preparations of of food for nutrition.

These are the most important basic rules of nutrition. Without those, everything is practically worthless.

Chapter 13

Bioenergy Body Balance Diet – BBB Diet

As the name says, the diet included is actually a healthy human diet with which the consumption of foods will be coordinated, and it leads to harmony or balance of the body. A foodstuff must also contain bioenergy. An example for that is unprocessed food. Processed foods will lose this benefit and properties. In this way, the requirements for the metabolic effect to happen will be fulfilled, and the combination of the food ingredients will be arranged in an optimal way.

Thus, the concerted and coordinated consumption of bioenergetic favorable foods will create conditions in the body for the free flow of bioenergy. In such circumstances, there is no energy blockage in the body, and the organs and metabolism are functioning in the best possible way. This leads to an optimal equilibrium or balance, so the person who nourishes him or herself upon the basic plan of the BBB Diet becomes and stays in equilibrium or balance. As a consequence, it will take about 12 weeks for the ideal weight of an individual to be realized.

Accordingly, the BBB Diet is a nutrition plan and is not a diet plan solely in terms of removing the excess weight, but a diet that will assist in achieving an ideal weight of an individual. This means that it also helps people who are malnourished to gain weight as much as it is optimal for their body type. This diet plan serves both groups of people, those who want to lose excessive pounds, and those who want to gain some weight. It is possible to achieve an ideal weight on a completely natural way, without any fasting or taking supplements for weight loss. And even better, the weight is maintained.

Who can benefit from the BBB Diet

The BBB Diet is suitable for all people, of all ages, and considers their body type. If you are pregnant, you are free to follow the BBB Diet plan, under condition that you are under the supervision of your doctor with whom you have spoken about taking calcium and/or Omega -3 supplements.

If you have diabetes, you can feel free to join the BBB Diet plan for nutrition, but you should have a regular medical checkup and measure your blood sugar levels before each meal. This is done in order to determine when and which snack you might consume in order that your blood sugar would not drop to a low value i.e. to hypoglycemia. As the time and approach of following the BBB Diet plan is anyway individual, there will be no need to change the schedule or the number of meals.

If you suffer from high blood pressure or some other illness, you can certainly follow a diet plan or one part of the plan that is convenient for you, in consultation with your physician.

It is certainly worth mentioning that in any kind of disease of an organ or the body, you should consult your physician or healthcare professional, which will discuss with you how to decide on a diet plan and what part of the BBB Diet is optimal for you.

The diet plan is set according to the ingredients and their quality, in order to facilitate the work of your vital organs, especially of the liver. It also enables you to increase your resistance and the function of the immune system. At the same time, a specific diet regime works in the prevention of the release of free radicals and decreases micro inflammatory processes in the body, which are slowing down the aging of the cells.

The BBB Diet plan will allow many of you to regulate high blood pressure or significantly reduce the risk of cardiovascular disease or diabetes type 2. Likewise, it will significantly reduce the risk of atherosclerosis, Alzheimer's disease and malignant tumors. This diet will benefit especially those who have difficulties with their liver and bile, whether it is the consequence of excessive alcohol consumption, virus infection, the consequence of drug use, HIV infection or malaria, intolerance to food and medicine, as well as people suffering from autoimmune diseases (i.e. Crohn's disease, ulcerative colitis, celiac disease).

The BBB Diet Guidelines

The BBB diet has no common rules according to which each person is supposed to nurture him or herself, because it is not possible to put that into operation. All those diets that contain general guidelines that apply to all persons are not effective, because they were not created to primarily determine which metabolic type of person you are.

Although planet Earth has about 7 billion different human beings, it is possible to talk about three different metabolic types, which are common for individuals. The science of Ayurveda was speaking about that thousands of years ago.

By such an approach previously described, the food is adjusted at the very beginning to a certain group of

individuals. With this systematic approach the optimal balance of nutrition is enabled.
What does it really mean? Simply put, this means that it matters when you eat, and how many times a day that you eat. Also, it is of course important what kind of food you consume, but also how is the food combined. It is quite confusing when talking about the daily food intake to hear or to read very often that you should divide your food into 5 meals. Everybody has probably heard about the "food pyramid". Some such plans are including 5 units of fruit daily, and 1-2 servings of salad and one serving of a vegetable. It is barely ever recommendable to consume five servings of fruit daily because of digestion or weight gain.

Try to keep a constant schedule of eating, respectively a timetable plan of your meals. This, however, does not mean that you need to practice excessive eating, just because it is time for your meal.

Do not eat too big of a portion because it burdens your part of the brain called the hypothalamus. The result is that the more you eat, the more you will have a need for food. Knowingly fruits are increasing cravings for food. But even without eating a single piece of fruit, by eating bigger portions, you will have a craving for more food.

Do not eat anything in-between meals, and especially

not fruits, because fructose or fruit sugar are exactly what the people, who tend to have a metabolic syndrome, are allowed to consume only in controlled quantity.
Also, you do not need to eat six times a day, i.e. almost every two hours. The body of an adult differs from a baby's body. You need to allow the body a certain time to digest and take a break from eating. This way you enable your digestion to be effective and balanced. The human body is a chemical factory that has its own law and order, and rules and regulations.

When you are in a chemical plant, you follow the rules. You respect the rules. Why not respect your own body? If you are eating every now and then, even if your organ functions are flawless, and you do not lack certain enzymes or components, this will result with chaos in the body. When and what you eat depends on your metabolic type and the type of diet you have chosen. This means that if you are, for example, a "pituitary metabolic type" or "adrenal metabolic type", you should eat a light breakfast that is consisting of vegetable juices with the addition of some Quinoa prepared the day before, some Chia-seeds with a spoon or two of fresh squeezed lemon juice.
Add to that a cup of coffee with no additives. And, that's all. You are ready to go to work and be fully concentrated until your lunchtime. You cannot eat all sorts of cereal with milk or yogurt, eggs, fruits, etc.,

because you do not have the metabolic conditions for that.

You cannot dig into breakfast just because it was called the most important meal of the day that needs to be plentiful and nourishing not to further repeat these constant mantras about proper nutrition.

If all your colleagues at work are having a snack, it does not mean that you should have one also, and that it would ok for you.

And finally, a proper and healthy diet for one person is not so for the other.

Getting ready for the Bioenergy Body Balance Diet

The BBB Diet is divided into 3 parts. The first part covers the first 7 days, the second part is the 3 weeks that follow thereafter, and the third part are individual meals and foods that can be added to the diet plan to maintain a constant weight. This third part takes two years to infinity. The body and metabolism will become so accustomed to the new way of eating during this period that the weight will not rollback. You will not have the same problems anymore that you had before you started reading this book regardless of what kind of problem we are talking about: whether there were aesthetic problems, medical problems or a combination of both.

For a diet you need a good and powerful blender and, if possible, one good quality juicer (the last is not a precondition).

The blender is used for food preparation of a paste called Hummus and a variety of thick juices for breakfast (smoothies). You need a juicer if you want to include vegetable juices for cleansing of the liver in your diet and to promote an adjustment toward a new way of eating.

With a little of organizing, you can prepare fresh juices and freeze them in 5 or 6 additional plastic cups in the freezer. This is the only way that every morning or before noon you can have an already prepared portion that will bring a positive effect in your diet without having to spend time cleaning your juicer. Juices that come from vegetables must be consumed fresh, but for most, the frozen option is the best method. Otherwise, you are falling into the habit of not consuming juices regularly due to lack of time.

You must be prepared for everything you do or intend to do, and so does your diet. You do not need to "physically" decide to do something good for your body, but rather mentally.

A diet is a change. Life after a diet is also a change. Ask yourself what it is that this change will bring to you. What kind of feeling will this change bring you afterwards? For example, if the answer to your question is that this change will bring you improvement of your health situation, ask yourself what would create this feeling of improvement: greater mobility, freedom, independence, peace of mind, greater understanding of the world around you, feeling of freedom and self-confidence, intense friendship with those around you, traveling, enjoying the food, new color of clothing that you wear, etc.

First you try to create conditions, which will enable you to be able to undertake profound thinking about the response that you are seeking from your subconscious. Do it while you are alone in a quiet place, where you will not be distracted or disturbed, for at least half an hour with pleasant music that is not too rhythmic or aggressive. Relax and sit back in the chair. You do not need necessarily to lie down, but you can if it suits you.

When you get the answer to your question, close your eyes and try to concentrate on a point that is located between the eyebrows, where the Hindus are having a colored spot on their forehead. Now try to calm down

and relax to allow your mind to create images of the response that you just have gotten. If your response is a greater sense of freedom, how are you experiencing it? What time of the year is it in front of your inner eye? Where exactly are you in this particular moment? What is the weather like? What time of day is it?
What colors can you notice around you? Are there any special odors? If your inner images through your thoughts have taken you on a travel, such as walking in the woods, by the lake, on a sandy beach, on a grassy meadow or in the mountains, let your inner "eye" see all the colors, to touch around and to smell. In short, let the images that are sliding in front of your third "eye" become a movie. You are free and very welcome to take part in this movie.

The next step is to try to create a plan, routine and discipline.

In order to "kick the old habits out of the saddle" that are so deeply rooted by certain behaviors and actions you must create a plan. These behaviors might be happening on a fully automatic basis, such as buying regularly at a certain time the croissants and pastries from the bakery around the corner. In psychology it is called "implementation of intention". You will be able to change these habits and achieve this step in your road toward your goal after reading the protocol of the BBB Diet.

The next step is to change your own routine as well as your habits. You do not want to get rid of the habits; you just want to change them.

Have you ever wondered and asked yourself, "What is a habit"? It is much easier to adopt and receive a benefit from if you know what it is. A habit is a choice of activities for which you have made the decision about at some point in time, and then it becomes second nature and is repeated constantly without thinking of what you are doing.

If you want to change your habits, you have to examine when and under what conditions your habit is happening, what you are doing over and over again, so that it has become your habit.

At the Massachusetts Institute of Technology, extensive studies have been conducted in 1990, which have shown the precision of the structure of human behavior known as a habit.

The study confirmed that the first step should be to analyze the structure of your present habits, so that they could be replaced by some new habits.

I will give you an example for this concerning the morning bagel purchase from the bakery around the corner. By this same principle you can make an exploration and analysis of any habit.

Let us start.

1. - Where are you at the moment when you deliberately decide to buy your bagel, as you do every morning? (You are in the bathroom.)
2. - What time is it? (It is 6:45 am.)
3. - What is your mood? (Actually, you are bored just like every other morning because you have to always repeat the same act. You are nervous as well because you are getting short of time)
4. - Who is in your surrounding area? (Nobody. You are alone.)
5. - What were you just about to do before you started thinking of rushing away? (You wanted to fix your hair? Your "roommate in your head" tell you that you are looking just fine the way you are. You want to check your mailbox on the computer but your "roommate" is telling you that you can do it at work. You want to drink the first cup of coffee but your inner voice is telling you that you can do it at the office as you are doing it every day while chatting with colleagues, etc.)

The next step then is to determine which of these conditions is forming your habit. Answer these questions every day during the next 5 days and write down the answers.

When does the certain pattern of an act happen? Is it when you do something that you must do every day the same way such as your morning hygiene. Therefore you have a need to think of something pleasant that you can do after your morning hygiene, which will then appear to you like a reward. Or is it rather too late to still be in the bathroom, so you have to speed up every day again and again and that way you are creating a stress for you every morning.

Or you are simply bored with the morning rituals? No one else is around? And the only thing you want is just to get to work and make your morning coffee with a bagel in company of others rather than being alone?

One of the responses will be repeated through all 5 days of testing.
In changing two of the five factors, you can change a habit.
For example:
* Get up a lot earlier in the morning to take care of the morning hygiene

* Start having showers regularly at night before bedtime

* Listen to the radio or television while preparing

yourself

* Spend 10 minutes every morning in a short exercise

* Make a decision the day before what are you going to have for breakfast and have your breakfast at home

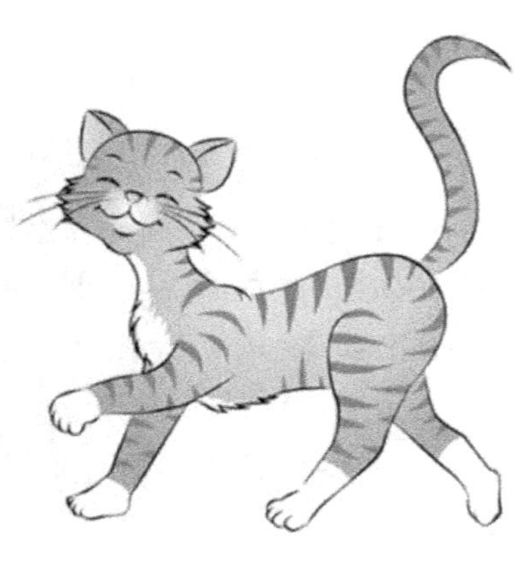

* For those who are alone, get yourself a cat. You will have multiple advantages. If you have a big family and you can afford it, get a dog and take a walk fifteen minutes in the morning before going to work, regardless of the weather.

* If you have a need for a morning coffee in the company of your colleagues, so do that. It is no need to have a bagel just because everybody else is having one.

Now what remains to be done is only to set out a plan,

consisting of the changes of those points that have led you to a particular habit. For example, drink a cup of coffee at home and eat a piece of Quinoa Cake (some delicious recipes can be found at the end the book). A complete book of recipes and foods for Bioenergy Body Balance with a number of recipes for simple unprocessed foods and healthy cooking, which will blow your mind, is expected to be published the end of 2013).

Try not to be too strict with yourself: if there are some days where you are still giving in to the old habits with a morning bagel on your way to work, observe the difference between these days, and those in which you acted upon your new plan. After some time you will determine that your mood was generally much better in the days when you have changed your habit, compared to days when you keep the old habits.

It will take some time until you can change and replace the habit. Your next step is that some of your habits should become rituals. Try, for example, to perform in the morning most of the things you do, the same way and at the same time. This will create a routine.

After that, you should get organized. This means that you can create in advance a plan for your weekly menu from morning to evening. Good organization, as in everything else in life, is a big part of success. Prepare a food protocol and a meals plan for the whole week, so that you don't need to think about groceries i.e. what to buy and what to eat.

In the first 7 days of the Diet hold the protocol and assemble your choice of foods without making any changes.

In the second week you can add a kind of food from your protocol list of foods as desired, but do not consume more than 3 meals with meat weekly. Ideally you should eat only fish three times a week. All sources of animal proteins, i.e. meat and fish, should be limited to a maximum of 200 grams daily. Daily intake of animal proteins for an adult is generally limited to 0.4 grams per pound of weight. This means that a normal adult weighting 140 pounds, who is not on a restricted diet, should consume no more than 56 grams of protein a day.

Your intake of proteins during the diet will be sufficient, and you will get more than enough proteins.

After the third part of the Diet, which means after 4 weeks, you can allow yourself to eat something in very reasonable quantities that does not belong to the diet and that is not recommended. You will realize that it means nothing to you and you find that this food is not so irresistible or tempting as it was before.

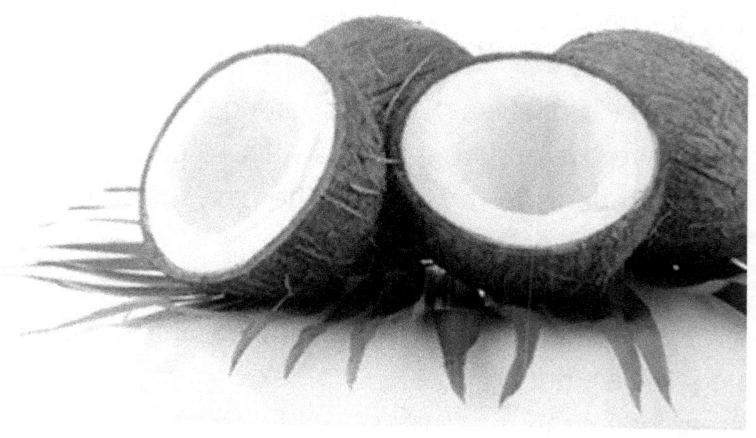

Protocol of the Bioenergy Body Balance Diet

1. The first week you should eat only vegetables. The exceptions are potatoes, cauliflower, beets, corn, and anything that contains starch and should not be consumed. Steamed vegetables should be consumed on a daily basis, except of those mentioned above. You should particularly choose all kinds of vegetables that have dark-green leaves such as kale, chard, collard greens, fennel (is good for digestion), and chicories (work well for function of bile).

Approximately 40% of the daily intake of vegetables should be in raw form. This includes all kinds of salads. If you have knowledge that you are poorly digesting all raw vegetables including salad, start chopping them into very thin strips and, and consume it prepared that way in small quantities. In addition, you can take one pill daily of a digestive enzyme.

In the first week, by not eating any meat or fish, you have the opportunity to switch to one of the types of vegetarianism. It would be the best thing you can do for your body.

You may consume an unlimited daily amount of vegetables during the first week, no matter whether steamed or raw.

The spices allowed are salt and pepper.

The dressing for all salads is exclusively made out of freshly squeezed lemon juice, 2-3 tablespoons of extra virgin olive oil, and salt and pepper.

Herbs are allowed.

Preferably consume fresh pressed garlic every day on your cooked vegetables. Garlic in the form of supplements, i.e. pills, is not having such a favorable absorption, as does fresh garlic, because the garlic contains the enzyme allicin, which is fully developing its effects in metabolic terms, 2 or 3 minutes after it has been chopped.

During the whole Diet you should use only natural sea salt in reasonable and rather moderate quantities.

Spices that are allowed for your cooked or steamed vegetables are sea salt, pepper and if you like it hot, Sambal Oelek (a chili pepper paste). If you are passionate in eating meat, only skinned poultry is allowed a maximum of 3 days a week. Fish consumed during the first week of the diet should be limited to tuna and salmon, preferably wild salmon, not farmed one.

Daily intake of meat or fish should be no more than 200 grams.

Fruits of any kind are not allowed in the first week with the exception of the juice of freshly squeezed lemons. Each morning begins with a glass of lukewarm water with fresh squeezed lemon juice. It is particularly good to add some lemon pulp to it because of digestion.

During the first two phases of the diet, which means the first 4 weeks, milk and dairy products should not be consumed in any form. This is of course including all kinds of cheeses.

Teas are allowed. However if you have a sensitive stomach and difficulties with digestion, you should void

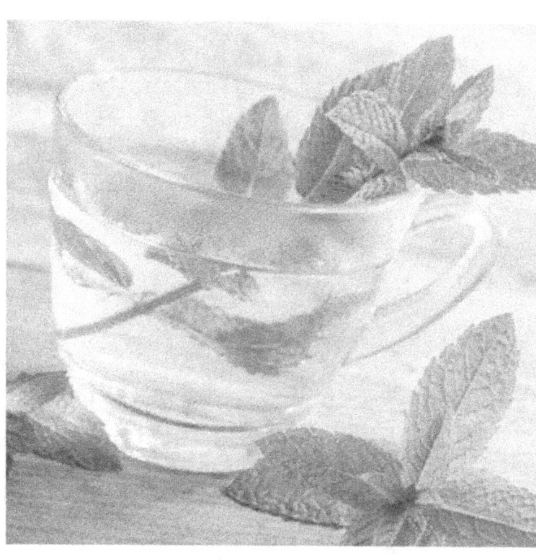

all green teas and teas based upon ethereal oils. The exception is the menthe tea. You should drink it during the summer months every day, hot and in small sips. If you have a chance, get yourself a dried leaf mint, which may be preserved and stored. Insert them into a cup of hot water or tea mug and allow the leaves to open. Otherwise, drink only organic teas of the best quality you can afford.

Black coffee is allowed in the morning as well as during the day. I recommend drinking filtered coffee of the best possible quality. Espresso coffee is pretty strong for the stomach lining, so if you like it, consumption should be limited to two cups daily.

For sweetening of your coffee or tea use Stevia.

Drink sparkling water or mineral water whenever you feel that you are thirsty. If it were recommendable to drink bottled water in the area where you live, a carbonated or sparkling water would be a better choice in this case.

Natural fruit juices are not allowed nor any kind of artificially sweetened drinks and sodas.

Drink vegetable juice freshly squeezed from the juicer every day.

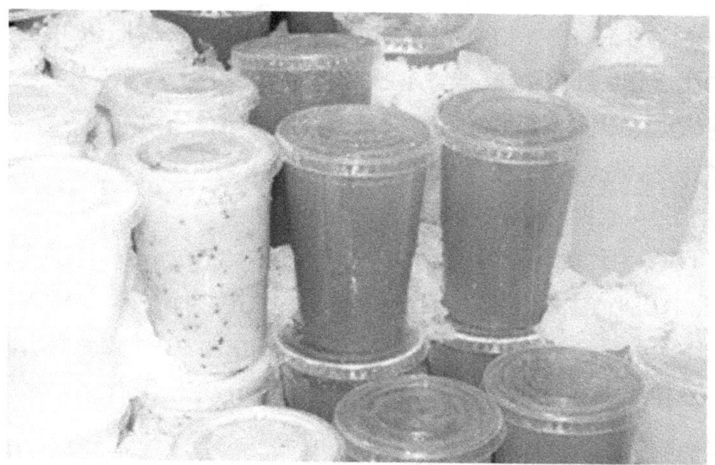

If you prepare a larger amount of juice once a week, and freeze it in plastic cups, you will have one cup for each day of the coming week.

Every day you can eat one hardboiled egg. However you can restrict your consumption of eggs to only one egg every 7 days, or leave it out completely, according to your taste.

2. In the second stage of the diet, i.e. after the first week, you might add a paste made out of chickpeas called Hummus. You can find the recipe for Hummus at the end of this book.

Hummus can be consumed for breakfast, and use fresh bell peppers, carrots and celery sticks cut into strips.

It is an ideal breakfast that gives plenty of energy for the whole morning.

Besides, you can consume Hummus during the day,

when you are having some other meal. Hummus is appropriate for any of three daily meals.

Cooked brown beans and kidney beans can be prepared on salad with onions, or simply with some organic virgin olive oil and salt.

There is no difference in the consumption of meat or fish whether in type or in quantity in the first week of the Diet: proteins of animal origin are allowed only 3 days a week and only a maximum of 200 grams per day.

Furthermore keep the habit of consuming a glass of water with lemon juice over the next 7 to 8 weeks. Lemon juice will neutralize the acid in the digestive system and create an alkali condition, and will be the driving force in cleansing of the liver.

You should drink daily homemade clear soup. The recipe can be found at the end of the book. For preparation you can use a steam pressure pot. The remaining soup can be stored in the refrigerator for 4 days or longer. Fresh cooked soup is also appropriate to be frozen. Soup can be prepared with only vegetables in the case that you are a vegetarian. Otherwise you can make it as a chicken soup by adding two larger pieces of chicken breast without skin to your soup recipe.

Pay attention to the total daily intake of animal protein. It is collective. If your soup contains chicken, you have consumed proteins of animal origin in liquid form. However it is recommended to consume soup almost every day.

Besides that, the soup will benefit your daily fluid intake, and will become a factor to strengthen your immune system.

Chop a peeled apple in a small processor daily. It takes you 5-7 seconds to grind it, and 3 minutes to clean the small processor. Scrubbing apples on a hand grinder does the same thing, but a small processor is indeed the fastest option. Then add the juice of half of one freshly squeezed lemon to the prepared apples. This can serve you as one whole meal if you drink a pint of soup after it.

Then again, be sure to combine those two meals only if the soup is a vegetable soup, with no chicken, since you should not eat fruits and proteins together.

Any kind of flour, preparations and the products made from flour and starch (cereals, rice, potatoes, pasta, and corn) are forbidden.

The next addition in this second phase is cashews and almonds. You can eat a dozen cashews and ten almonds a day.

At this stage of the diet it is allowed to prepare vegetables in a Wok. It is convenient to prepare frozen vegetables except cauliflower, eggplant and corn, which are sometimes in the frozen mixture. Be aware of this when purchasing. When preparing your vegetables in a Wok, the allowed spices are salt, pepper and a little of clear soup with vegetables and chicken, which can be added to the Wok dish at the end of cooking.

All soy sauces and all soy products are prohibited during the diet. This is because 8 out of 10 people are having problems with irritations of the gut because of the soy products. It is also known as a Chinese restaurant syndrome.

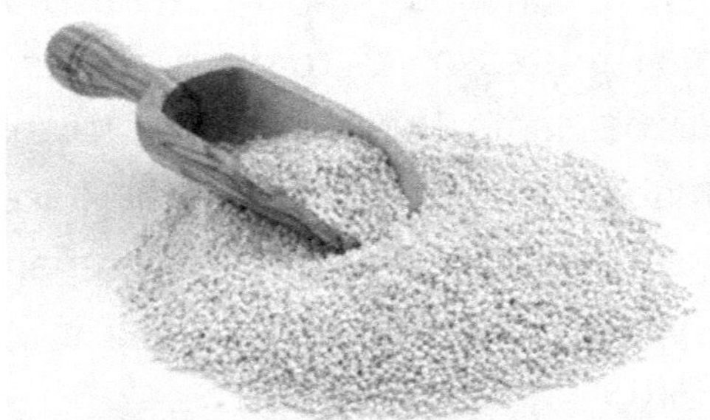

The following food that will be pleasurable and fill you up with energy is Quinoa. It is the seed of a plant that belongs to the family of Swiss chard, and is cultivated in the Andes in Peru at an altitude of 3,000 meters. In Peru, where it is a main export product, Quinoa has become a monoculture.

It contains the highest percentage of protein among plants. One cup (125 ml) Quinoa contains 9 g of protein, which is much better absorbed in the body than milk protein (casein). In addition it is important to say that Quinoa can be enjoyed without limitation, because it has no gluten.

Quinoa is the only source of all 9 amino acids in the vegetable world.

Incas consumed Quinoa as one of the main sources of food over 6000 years ago.

Quinoa may be prepared in various ways and eaten

cold or warm, salty or sweet. The basic recipe for cooking Quinoa is at the end of the book.

3. The third part of the diet takes place from the fourth week onwards. If you have come so far, I hope you have adopted a new way of eating which should contribute to an ideal balance of the entire body. It will also contribute to ideal weight.

After the fourth week, feel free to start adding some fruit to your Diet according to your taste and preferences.

It is not out of the ordinary to bring up, that it is good to give priority to the seasonal fruit. The best kinds of fruits are cherries, pink grapefruit, plums, bananas (which you can also use for your morning shake), blueberries (preferred are natural ones, not cultivated) and raspberries.

Exotic fruits, such as pineapple, papaya or mango are having great advantages, because they contain valuable enzymes for digestion, but are otherwise having a high GI index.

All the meals and products with starch, flour, and pasta should be at best not consumed at all or reduced to a minimum. There are people who eat very little bread. And then there are others who enjoy it, in all ways and always. They don't care if the bread is fresh or old.

The person of the last group is addicted to the bread and should completely stop to consume the bread, because they are not able to get satisfied with only one or two slices.

If you have decided to include bread in your diet, choose to eat only rye bread or bread made of Dinkel flour, which is made from hulled wheat. However, this flour contains gluten. If you cannot consume gluten, then you may choose any form of gluten-free flour, which unfortunately has a higher content of carbohydrates. If you decide not to completely exclude flour out of your menu, a good substitute is one flour tortilla a day. The advantage lies certainly in the homemade tortilla, and not the purchased one.

Even if you are short on time, you can prepare Tortillas in larger quantities and store them in the refrigerator in plastic wrap.

This way you can use the flour of your choice.

The recipe for preparation of homemade tortillas can be found at the end of the book.

You can occasionally add to your Diet dishes with a sweet potato. One simple but very tasty recipe you will find at the end of this book.

4. Do not mix and combine proteins with fruits in the same meal in your nutrition. A time break between the two of those should be at least 2 hours.

In order to be digested, proteins need an entirely different enzyme and amino acid than those for the digestion of fruits. If you consume protein and fruits in the same meal, it will be fermented and you are making a small winery out of your stomach, due to fermentation. Proteins therefore start to rot in the stomach before digestion can be initiated.

5. Give preference to drinking bottled water, although a tap water is ok when it is of a good quality.

The plastic material of the bottles is not exactly the healthiest choice, but in the lack of glass bottles, you'll

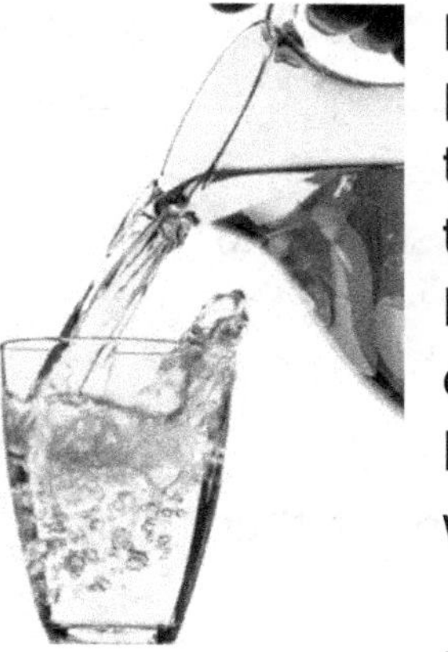

probably reach for water from a plastic bottle. And if you do so, then rather have sparkling water than just a still mineral water, because the risk of contamination after opening the bottle is smaller by sparkling water.

Ordinary tap water contains, to be precise, fluorine and chlorine, which are inhibiting the absorption of iodine.

6. The salad dressings should be made only out of fresh squeezed lemon juice, organic virgin olive oil and sea salt.

Avoid all kinds of vinegar, whether it is wine vinegar or fruit vinegar, for the reasons I have described previously.

If you don't want to give up on vinegar, then your safest choice is Umiboshi vinegar. This vinegar is produced from fruit growing in Japan that can be described as a merge between a plum and apricot. The

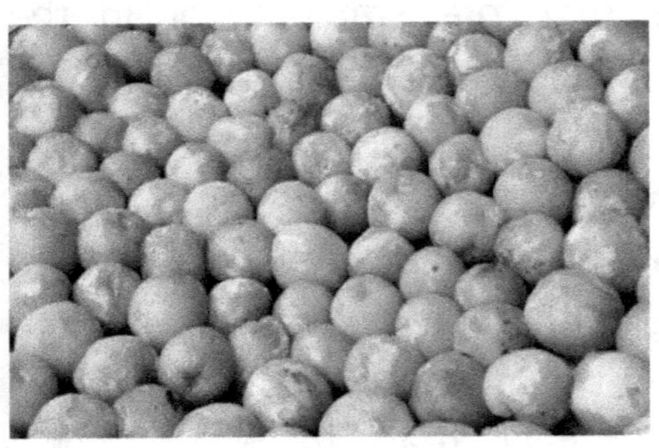

Umiboshi is 20% salt and acid, and it is antibacterial and antitoxic. It is consumed not only as vinegar, but also dried as an Apéro-snack. A health tonic that is good for digestion, especially the digestion of rice is made out of the green Ume fruits.

In Japan there is a saying similar to ours in the Western world: one apple a day, keeps the doctor away - the same is said for the Ume.

Beverages prepared from the Ume were given to the samurai before battle, to protect them from being tired.

7. Eat seaweed. This "sea lettuce" has a beneficial effect in lowering cholesterol and blood pressure. It contains Potassium, Magnesium, Iron and Manganese and it has traces of 60 different minerals. Besides, it is the only plant that is a source of vitamin B12. Seaweed has also antibacterial and anti radioactive properties. It has been proven by an experiment at the University of McGill in Montreal, Canada. They made extensive scientific tests on aliginic acid, which is contained in seaweed.

One large group of physicians and their patients

survived the effects of the atomic bomb on Hiroshima in Japan by regularly eating seaweed.

Best-known seaweeds are Wakame and Nori. Most of the time you can get those at the grocery departments that are selling fresh fish.

8. Eat Avocado regularly, at least twice a week. You can prepare it simply sliced on a salad or smashed with a fork into a paste. To do so, the avocado must be soft but still bright green, so it can be mixed together with salt, lemon, garlic and olive oil. A recipe for this delicious paste is at the end of the book.

It is wonderful with fish or chicken. The paste can be stored up to one week in the refrigerator in a good closed glass jar.

The Avocado contains vitamins such as C, E and B6, and is rich in calcium, copper and the fibrin fibers.

Avocado lowers cholesterol and high blood pressure. It has been proven that its component *glutathion* is preventing colon cancer.

9. A Swiss chard should be on your weekly menu in the months when there is plenty of it, i.e. spring through autumn.

It is very delicious steamed with garlic, and spiced with sea salt, pepper and virgin olive oil.

A Swiss chard contains calcium, magnesium and fibrin fibers. It is participating actively against lung inflammation and as prevention against the formation

of pulmonary emphysema if consumed regularly.
Besides, Swiss chard is preventing colon cancer and prostate cancer.

It is widely known that the chard as well as kale is an indispensable part of Mediterranean cuisine.
Less known is that one cup of Swiss Chart (250 ml) contains as much calcium as a 7 ounce glass of milk.

10. Get used to eating a fresh raw bell pepper every day. The best ones are those of red color, because they contain the most of the vitamin C.

In addition to the vitamins C, A, B, and E, bell peppers contain beta-carotene, which is working against inflammation, and *Capsacain*, a substance that lowers cholesterol and is working very powerfully in the prevention of diabetes.

The content of sulfur in the peppers works against cancer, whereby *lutein* prevents building of the eye cataracts and macular degeneration of the eye.

11. The choice of all kinds of salads is really plentiful in the summer, and I am sure that many of you are enjoying this colorful, refreshing and tasty meal.

But I want to draw your attention specially to the salad that contains red fleshy peppers, onions, tomatoes and cucumbers chopped into very small cubes and seasoned properly with standard dressing for the salad: sea salt, lemon and olive oil. In Israel, you can get it packed into plastic containers with the dressing mentioned on side under the name- Israeli salad.

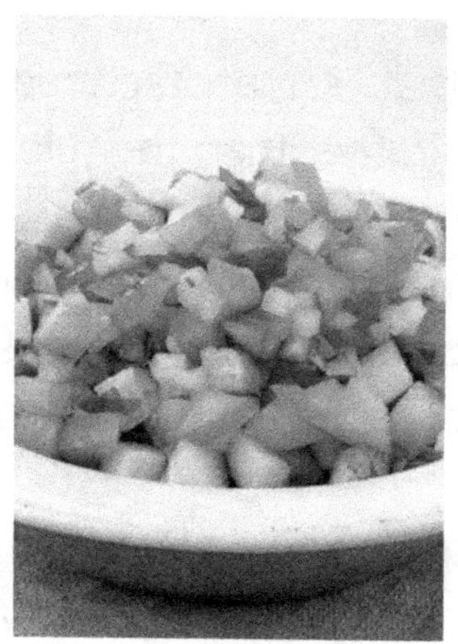

It has several benefits at the same time. It is good for digestion, because it is very finely cut, it satisfies the thirst, and it is refreshing and has all you need in one meal.

Similar or almost the same salad is served in India under the name Kachumber.

12. Never consume anything that is sweetened with artificial sweeteners.

If a person has a disorder called Fatty liver, it is better to ask him or her if they are consuming artificially sweetened drinks rather then to ask them about their alcohol consumption.

If the NAFLD (nonalcoholic fatty liver disease) does not get cured or taken care of, it can evolve into liver cirrhosis.

Another equally important and bad consequence of artificially sweetened drinks is your teeth. Almost all cavities by young patients that I have dealt with were connected with artificial and regular soda consumption. All of those patients had cavities on open teeth surfaces or a general massive prevalence of cavities that I was able to define with their eating habits. It has to be underlined that all sodas are having a negative impact, because of their content of phosphoric acid that will erode tooth enamel (General Dentistry, 2007)

13. Try not to consume food that is manufactured. If you must, let it be the exception rather than the rule.

14. Consume fruits within certain limits. After consumption the fruit does not create the substances Leptin and Ghrelin, which are responsible for satiety, so that a person keeps on eating. In addition a person's appetite is rising after eating fruits. It has been proven by scientific study of the scientists Shapiro, MD / Ph.Scarpace, MD, from the University of Florida, USA.

The people that are constantly eating fruit are producing the enzyme *fructocinase* mostly in large quantities.

This enzyme works in the body as a transporter of the glucoses from the intestine further into the blood. Many people are not properly splitting fructose. Instead, bacteria are breaking down fructose i.e. fruit sugar, that is leading to the formation of gas. At that point, the person can feel bloated or uncomfortable. If the reaction is stronger, this same process is starting to pull water from the gut, which leads to diarrhea.

The drug for inhibition of fructocinase will surely be invented sooner or later. For now, you can keep the consumption of fruits under control, or choose not to eat fruits at all.

If you are regularly consuming fructose and fruits, then you need to stop your consumption every 6 months for a period of up to 2 weeks, to allow the level of the enzyme to get back to normal.

The intensive researches, that are still ongoing for disease of IBS Irritable bowel syndrome, have shown that these people have a disturbance in fructose absorption. (University of Iowa)

It has to be especially brought to your attention to stay away from a widespread consumption of orange juice for one more reason: orange juice reduces the hardness of your teeth.

15. Use *turmeric* spice on a daily basis. Turmeric is a spice whose beneficial and distinctive properties have been known for thousands of years in Chinese and Indian medicine.

Turmeric spice is sold in pulverized form, and it can be very easily added to all kind of different dishes like salads, soups, vegetables and fish.

By purchasing turmeric, you should certainly give advantage to pure organic turmeric without any add-ons.

The active substance in turmeric is called *Curcumin*. It is most effective if turmeric is used in its natural, original form. Capsules of curcumin that is attainable, as supplements are not absorbed as successfully in the body as the natural spice.

Turmeric has a strong effect in suppressing inflammation in the body, which is, as I mentioned earlier, one of the main causes of chronic diseases. Turmeric works also in combating cancer.

In the scientific work performed by Brazilian scientists, which has been published in June 2012, it was proven in the in vitro experiments that turmeric was able to suppress one of the most evil brain cancer cells (glioblastoma), without harming the normal cells.

Besides, turmeric has been proven as inhibitor of other kind of cancer cells such as lung cancer and prostate cancer.

It is also known that turmeric is involved in the processes of more than 500 genes in the human body.

16. Use lemons in your diet all day along, from morning to evening.

The lemon might be consumed by adding it into water, dressings, and sauces, on steamed vegetables, fish and broth. Lemons are not only having the power to alkalize the body, but are also reducing salt in the food that we consume.

When purchasing, choose your lemons with a thinner and smoother peel because they contain more juice. Wash them well and roll them with a palm on a hard surface to allow the juice to be divided inside of the fruit. Now, it is ready to cut.

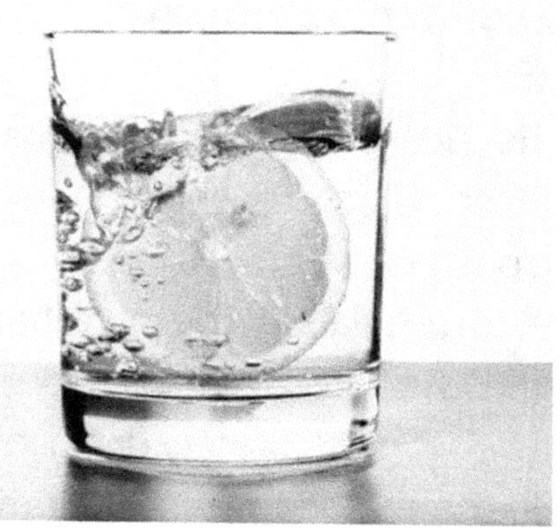

Do not consume pure lemon juice undiluted, because it is damaging for the enamel on the teeth.

Further, a lemon has positive properties because of its high content of vitamin C and is having beneficial effects on the liver, gallbladder, and intestines and is lowering the uric acid in the body.

Beside these healing properties, the lemon has a beneficial effect on the lungs and breathing under physical exertion. An example for this is the statement of the first conqueror of Mt. Everest, Edmund Hillary, who said that he owes lemons credit for assisting him with his spectacular climb.

17. Use natural organic cinnamon powder. It is important to consume it regularly, because it has a significant impact on the metabolism of sugar. Get your cinnamon powder from Ceylon, which is an island in the West Indies and has the best possible quality.

It is very convenient to consume it with your morning coffee

Cinnamon is not only the spice for apples; it is widely used in cooking, an example of which is the unusually delicious Moroccan cuisine.

In addition to regulating the metabolism of sugar, cinnamon has other medicinal properties such as lowering the level of cholesterol, disabling the bacteria H. pylori that is the major causes of stomach ulcers, as well as stops many other pathogenic bacteria.

Besides being a natural preservative, cinnamon acts against arthritic pain, and scientific studies have attributed to it anticancer and medicinal properties to combat neurodegenerative diseases such as Alzheimer D., Parkinson's D., multiple sclerosis and meningitis. This is published in scientific studies of Cytokine Research Laboratory, Department of Experimental Therapeutics,
University of Texas.

18. Include fats in your diet.

The human body requires fat in order to function normally. So there is no question that including fat in your diet is essential, but the question is what kind of fat is useful and what kind of fat you should not consume.

Use whenever possible the best quality virgin olive oil.

It is perfect as a condiment, but is tolerating on the

other hand only a low cooking temperature.

Cut out eating all saturated oils and fats, especially those of dense consistency saturated fats, such as margarines and toppings. These are all the fats that are produced in a process of hydrogenation.

The only exception of saturated fat that is recommended for consumption is pure organic coconut oil, which can be used for cooking of food at high temperatures.

Coconut oil is not only helping you lose your weight because it helps absorption of the essential fatty acids in the body, but it is as well the only fat that does not develop harmful ingredients by heating i.e. so called trans-fats, which raise the value of CRP (C-reactive protein). The CRP is the most important measurement and indicator of inflammation in the body.

In smaller quantities consume *Ghee*, which has been used in the science of Ayurveda for thousands of years as a food and as an application for the skin in variety of forms and preparations.

The ghee is made out of butter in a simple manner, in that the butter is warmed on a very low temperature, which separates the butter fat from scum that is collected on the surface. It is casein, i.e. milk protein and lactose, i.e. milk fat.

It is important to use only pure organic butter of the best quality for the preparation of the ghee.

So prepared, ghee can be stored in the refrigerator

in a small porcelain container up to 3 weeks.

19. Make sure that your teeth and mouth hygiene are included in a regular care, control and recall program of your dentist at least once a year.

The teeth are the mirrors of your body.

Make sure you learn how to properly clean your teeth and oral cavity and do not miss the daily ritual of mouth and teeth hygiene under any circumstances.

Your goal is that your teeth are taken care of in the way that you do not have to have significant procedures that are required for a longer period of time.

More on this topic can be found in my next book on BBB-Diet and nutrition, which is coming out at the end of 2013.

20. Living a diet, which ensures the balanced functioning of your entire body, you do not need necessarily to count calories, but it is important to limit the total daily intake of food. As a measure, after Phase 2 of the diet, you can use one shallow plate of 10.5 inches and fill it up with cooked foods of your choice that you will be eating during that day. It can be cooked food, raw food, cooked meat, fish or eggs.

This excludes breakfast and everything that you consume in a liquid form.

You can overload your plate, but this is the daily quantity of foods that you may eat that day. It does not matter if you will consume that big plate of food at once, or you are going to split it into several meals in one day.
As I mentioned before, do not eat more than 2 or maximum 3 meals a day.

The quantity of liquids or liquid food is not limited, so you may have all the homemade vegetable soup (with or without chicken) that you want.

Chapter 14

Recipes

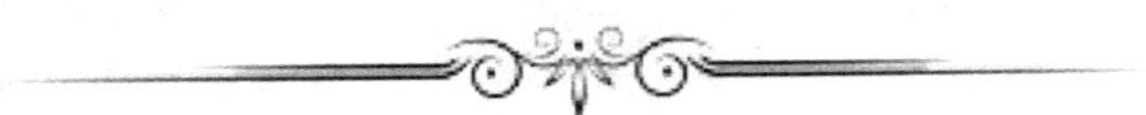

Vegetable soup (optionally with chicken)

The quantity is meant for a pressure steam pot of 6 liters or 1.5 gallons. Cooking time is about 1.5 hours.

If you want to cook your soup in an ordinary pot, then you have to cook it slow removing the foam from the top of the soup regularly. Cooking time is 4 hours.

Ingredients:

1 bunch of parsley
1 piece of celery root, size of one small apple
2 pieces of stick celery
2 large carrots
1/4 head of cabbage
1 onion
2 garlic cloves
1 parsley root
1 piece of pealed ginger, size of a plum
1 tea container filled halfway with pepper kernels

2 cubes of Maggi Chicken *Bouillon Cube* or vegetable soup (it can be any other brand but be sure to choose a product without E-numbers or additives)
1 small tomato
2 tablespoons genuine sea salt
2 pcs. Chicken breast without skin

Filtered broth can be stored in the refrigerator or freezer in portions.

Breakfast

This breakfast is prepared in a mixer. You can decide yourself on a consistency, adjusting the water. This is the basic recipe for one person.

Ingredients:

1 peeled apple
1/2 cup cooked Quinoa (125 ml)
1/2 fresh squeezed lemon-juice
1 small amount of cinnamon powder measured on the tip of a knife

If you would like a sweeter juice, you can use a teaspoon of honey or a few drops of Stevie will do.

In the third stage of the diet, i.e. after 4 weeks, you

can add half of a banana or
very few of other seasonal fruit to add the flavor.

Try to experiment with flavors and your imagination will have no limits.

If you add one beaten egg to the basic ingredients, without adding any water, dough can be made and baked in a primed baking pan (organic coconut oil). You'll get an incredibly yummy cake, which you can carry to work.

Hummus

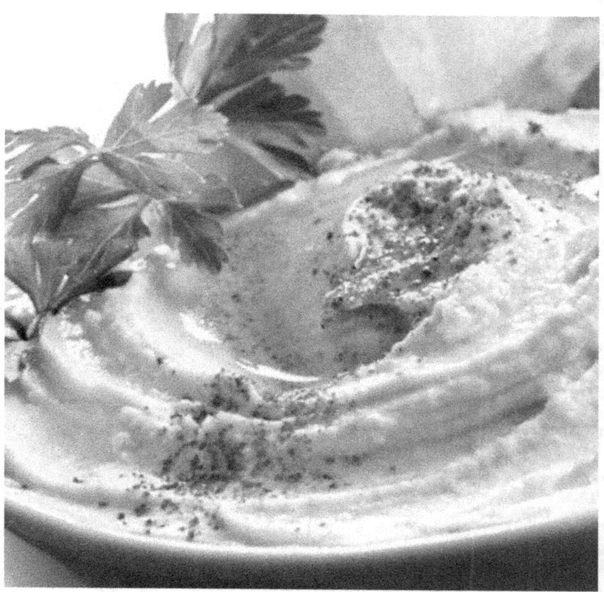

This nourishing paste is served cold, thinly smeared on a shallow plate, sprinkled with red pepper powder and a little extra virgin olive oil on the surface. In my opinion it is an excellent dish and cannot be beaten, whether in the nutrition nor in the taste. It is matchless and supreme.

Hummus can be enjoyed and served from morning until

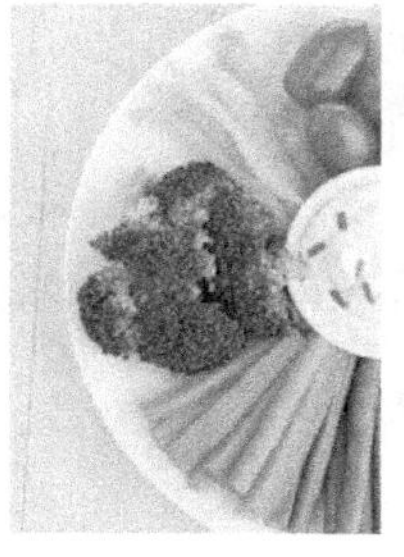

evening: as a lunch, appetizer, snack or a dinner. It is normally served with vegetables cut into sticks. In the Middle East, where from the paste originated, it is traditionally served with pita bread. I suppose that many of you enjoy Hummus bought at the grocery store, and it is not bad, but what is so exciting about it? Just try homemade Hummus prepared upon the recipe below and you will get the answer.

Ingredients:

500 g (2 cups) chickpeas beans (canned or self cooked)
2 tablespoons Tahina paste (paste made from sesame seeds and oil)
2 lemons
2 cloves of garlic
1 ml (1/4 of a teaspoon) of water (depending on the quantity of the lemon juice)
1 teaspoon sea salt
white pepper powder

The canned chickpeas should be thoroughly washed, put in a bowl of cold water to soak. Remove the transparent membrane with the fingers. To make this easier you might soak them in the water overnight. Squeeze two lemons and only the juice will be used. Add all the prepared ingredients into the mixer and blend at a strong setting. The paste should have a consistency that is solid and sticky, and not liquid. Add water to achieve the desired consistency.

Hummus can be refrigerated in a tightly sealed glass container 4-5 days.

Quinoa

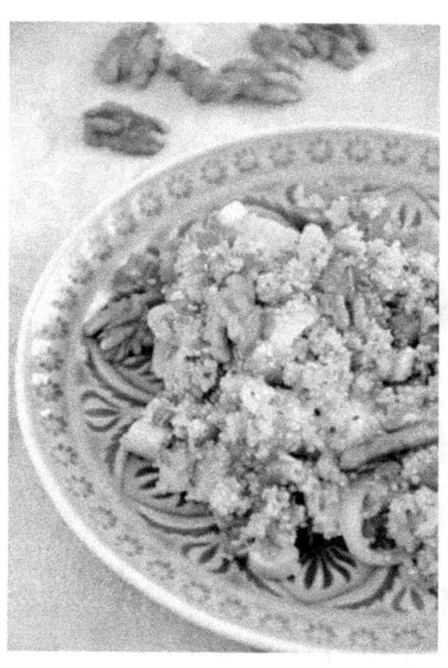

Washed Quinoa seeds are cooked 20 minutes in lightly boiling water, clear vegetable soup or chicken soup.

The quantity is one measure of Quinoa and 2.5 measures of the liquid.
After cooking, Quinoa should rest on the stove to get a firm dish.

The Year 2013 has been proclaimed by the United Nations as the year of Quinoa.

Sweet potatoes

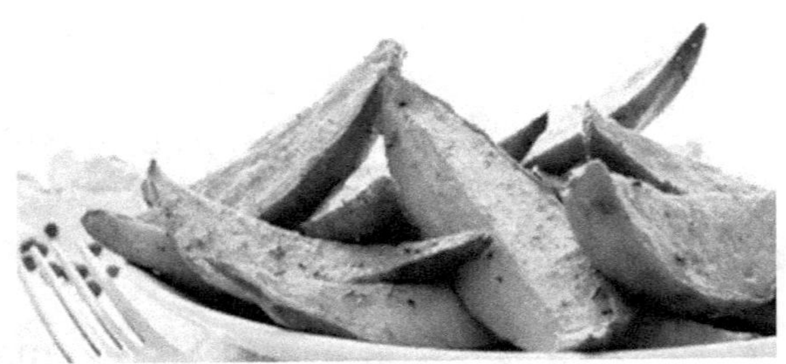

Peel the potatoes so that an intense orange color is visible.

Cut lengthwise into eighths (depending on size of potatoes) and place in a bowl and sprinkle with sea salt. Stir well.

Put the potatoes into an ovenproof dish and bake in a preheated oven at 220°C or 425°F. Cook until the potatoes begin to gently rumple and the edges are starting to get brown.

Serve immediately.

Avocado Paste

The measure refers to 1 piece of avocado. Quantities can certainly be multiplied. The paste can be well preserved in small glass jars in the refrigerator.

Ingredients:

1 avocado
1 clove garlic
sea salt for the taste
1 tablespoon freshly squeezed lemon juice
2 tablespoons extra virgin olive oil

The consistency of the avocado must be so soft that it is mashable with a fork. Mince the garlic and smear it with a knife into the paste adding some sea salt. Add the already crushed avocado, taste and add some more salt if needed.

Next, stir in fresh squeezed lemon juice, stirring until the paste is smooth, and finally stir in the olive oil with same movements.

Tortilla

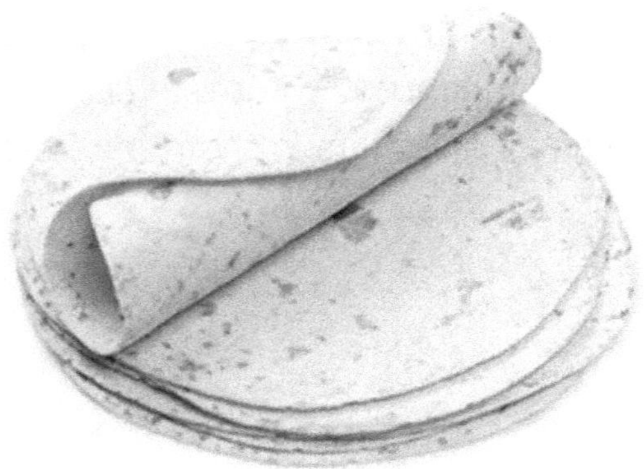

The measure gives a quantity of 10 to 12 Tortillas. The advantage of preparing homemade tortillas is that you can define the choice of flour yourself.

Moreover, that way you are sure that there are no additional processed food preservatives inside of your Tortilla.

Ingredients:

2 cups (500 ml) of flour
1/2 teaspoon salt
1/4 cup (50 ml) of flaxseed oil
1/2 cup (125 ml) to 3/4 cup (175 ml) warm water
1 tablespoon baking powder

Mix flour (for example Dinkel or other dark flour of smooth consistency, with no seeds or sprouts, NO corn flour) with salt and baking powder.

Add the oil, then stir and mix with your fingers slowly adding water. Consistency must be adhesive, so that you can form a sticky ball.

Wrap dough ball in plastic wrap and let it stand for 30 minutes.

Remove the plastic wrap, form out of one dough ball 8 smaller balls and cover them with a clean cloth or towel that has been heated over warm steam or in steamer.

Roll the dough balls on a floured surface while hot - otherwise the dough will be tough. Always fold the dough in half while rolling, and then fold it again and again, repeating it a dozen times, until the dough has a thin round shape.

Bake in heavy pan with oil that is pretty hot. The best thing to do is to use a pure organic virgin coconut oil.

Bake each tortilla in a large heavy pan from each side for about 30 seconds. Place each tortilla immediately in the preheated hot steamed towel.

Let the tortillas pile up for a while under the hot

steamed fabric cloth allowing them to cool down.

Place them in a plastic bag without folding them and seal the bag well. The tortillas may be stored in a refrigerator without a problem for sure over 1 week.

Links

1. http://www.WebMD.com

2. http://www.Mayoclinic.com

3. http://www.Lumosity.com

4. http://bioenergieheilung.ch

5. http://www.hypnosetherapie-schweiz.ch

6. http://holisticka-energija.com.hr/en/

7. Behaviorally conditioned immunosuppression - http://www.psychosomaticmedicine.org/content/37/4/333.abstract

8. Functional Links between the Immune System, Brain Function and Behavior - http://grants.nih.gov/grants/guide/pa-files/pa-05-054.html

9. Biochemical Aspects of Anxiety - http://www.ncbi.nlm.nih.gov/books/NBK28190/

10. Kosher salt - http://en.wikipedia.org/wiki/Kosher_salt

11. Hypnosetherapie - http://www.hypnosetherapie-schweiz.com/

References

Chapter 1.

R Ader and N Cohen. Behaviorally conditioned immunosuppression. Psychosomatic Medicine, Vol 37, Issue 4 333-340

Elenkov IJ, Iezzoni DG, Daly A, Harris AG, Chrousos GP. "Cytokine dysregulation, inflammation and well-being". Neuroimmunomodulation. 2005;12(5):255-69

Leserman, J., Jackson, E. D., Petitto, J. M., Golden, R. N., Silva, S. G., Perkins, D. O., Cai, J., Folds, J. D., and Evans, D. L. (1999). Progression to AIDS: the effects of stress, depressive symptoms, and social support. Psychosomatic Medicine 61(3), 397-

Zorrilla, E. P., Luborsky, L., McKay, J. R., Rosenthal, R., Houldin, A., Tax, A., McCorkle, R., Seligman, D. A., & Schmidt, K. (2001). The relationship of depression and stressors to immunological assays: a meta-analytic review. Brain Behavior and Immunity, 15(3), 199-226.

McDonald RD, Yagi K. A note on eosinopenia as an index of psychological stress. Psychosom Med 1960;2 22: 149–50.

Chapter 2.

Cowen, Richard (May 1999). "The Importance of Salt". UC Davis Department of Geology.

Gary Taubes (2 June 2012). "Salt, We Misjudged You". *The New York Times*.

Chapter 3.

Zinn-Justin, Jean; *Quantum Field Theory and Critical Phenomena,* Oxford University Press (2002)

O'Brien, Paul (2007). *Divination: Sacred Tools for Reading the Mind of God.* Visionary Networks Press

Wilhelm, R. & Baynes, C., (1967): "The I Ching or Book of Changes", with foreword by Carl Jung, Introduction, Bollingen Series XIX, Princeton University Press, (1st ed. 1950)

Lao Zi: Tao Te Ching

Robson, T (2004). *An Introduction to Complementary Medicine.* Allen & Unwin. pp. 90

Deadman, P; Baker K; Al-Khafaji M (2007). *A Manual of Acupuncture.* Journal of Chinese Medicine Publications

Chapter 4.

Tipler, Paul (2004). *Physics for Scientists and Engineers: Electricity, Magnetism, Light, and Elementary Modern Physics*

Chapter 5.

"About Nikola Tesla". Tesla Memorial Society of NY. Retrieved 5 July 2012.

"Tesla Quotes". Tesla universe. Retrieved 5 July 2012.

[About Nikola Tesla "About Nikola Tesla"]. Tesla Society of USA and Canada. Retrieved 5 July 2012.

Seifer, Marc J. (1998). *Wizard the life and times of Nikola Tesla : biography of a genius*. Secaucus, N.J.: Citadel Press/Kensington Publishing Corp..

New York Herald Tribune, 11 September 1932

"THE PROBLEM OF INCREASING HUMAN ENERGY". Twenty-First Century Books. Retrieved 21 April 2011.

Meyl, Konstantin, H. Weidner, E. Zentgraf, T. Senkel, T. Junker, and P. Winkels, *Experiments to proof the evidence of scalar waves Tests with a Tesla reproduction*. Institut für Gravitationsforschung (IGF),

Am Heerbach 5, D-63857 Waldaschaff.

T.R.Swartz: " The Last Journals of Nikola Tesla: Haarp - Chemtrails and Secret of Alternative 4 "

N. Tesla: The Fantastic Inventions of Nikola Tesla, 1993

Hooper, Dan (2006). *Dark Cosmos: In Search of Our Universe's Missing Mass and Energy*. New York: HarperCollins

Smolin, Lee (2006). *The Trouble with Physics: The Rise of String Theory, the Fall of a Science, and What Comes Next*. New York: Houghton Mifflin

Susskind, Leonard (2006). *The Cosmic Landscape: String Theory and the Illusion of Intelligent Design*. New York: Hachette Book Group/Back Bay Books.

1. Thomas C. Martin: Inventions, Researches and Writings of Nikola Tesla

Chapter 6.

Neuropeptides and Other Bioactive Peptides: From Discovery to Function, L.D.Fricker, Morgan & Claypool Publishers, 2012

Elias A. Said *et al.* 2009, PD-1 Induced IL10 Production by

Monocytes Impairs T-cell Activation in a Reversible Fashion" *Nature Medicine* 2010; 452-9.

Bruce, Robert: *Auric Mechanics and Theory*, "Capturing the Aura," pp 301-303. Blue Dolphin Publishing, 2000

Breaux, *Journey Into Consciousness: The Chakras, Tantra and Jungian Psychology*, Motilal Banarsidass, 1998

Taylor Latener, Rodney Leon (2005). *The Illustrated Encyclopedia of Confucianism, Vol. 2*. New York: Rosen Publishing Group.

Hoopes, Aaron (2007). *Zen Yoga: A Path to Enlightenment though Breathing, Movement and Meditation*. Kodansha International.

Plotkin SA (April 2005). "Vaccines: past, present and future". *Nature Medicine* **11** (4 Suppl): S5–11.

Medzhitov R (October 2007). "Recognition of microorganisms and activation of the immune response". *Nature* **449** (7164): 819–26

Kawai T, Akira S (February 2006). "Innate immune recognition of viral infection". *Nature Immunology* **7**

Flower DR, Doytchinova IA (2002). "Immunoinformatics and the prediction of immunogenicity". *Applied Bioinformatics* **1**

Langley-Evans SC, Carrington LJ (2006). "Diet and the

developing immune system".

Bryant PA, Trinder J, Curtis N (June 2004). "Sick and tired: Does sleep have a vital role in the immune system?". *Nature Reviews. Immunology*

Leif Mosekilde (2005). "Vitamin D and the elderly". *Clinical Endocrinology*

Hertoghe T (December 2005). "The 'multiple hormone deficiency' theory of aging: is human senescence caused mainly by multiple hormone deficiencies?". *Annals of the New York Academy of Sciences*

Chandra RK (August 1997). "Nutrition and the immune system: an introduction". *The American Journal of Clinical Nutrition*

Watts, Alan. "11 _10-4-1 Meditation." *Eastern Wisdom: Zen in the West & Meditations.* The Alan Watts Foundation. (2009)

University of Wisconsin-Madison (2008, March 27). Compassion Meditation Changes The Brain. ScienceDaily.

Goleman, Daniel (1988). *The meditative mind: The varieties of meditative experience*. New York:

Zen Buddhism : a History: India and China by Heinrich Dumoulin, James W. Heisig, Paul F. Knitter (2005)

Soto Zen in Medieval Japan by William Bodiford (2008)
B. Rael Cahn & John Polich (2006). "Meditation states and traits: EEG, ERP, and neuroimaging studies". *Psychological Bulletin* (American Psychological Association) (2): 180–211.

Dunne and Davidson, "Meditation and the Neuroscience of Consciousness: An Introduction" in *The Cambridge handbook of consciousness* by Philip David Zelazo, Morris Moscovitch, Evan Thompson, (2007)

Austin, James H. (1999) *Zen and the Brain: Toward an Understanding of Meditation and Consciousness*, Cambridge: MIT Press,

Bennett-Goleman, T. (2001) *Emotional Alchemy: How the Mind Can Heal the Heart*, Harmony Books

Shalif, Ilan et al. (1989) *Focusing on the Emotions of Daily Life* (Tel-Aviv: Etext Archives, 2008)

Sogyal Rinpoche, *The Tibetan Book of Living and Dying*,

Oldstone-Moore, Jennifer. *Understanding Confucianism*, Duncan Baird, (2003)

Harper, Donald; Michael Loewe and Edward L. Shaughnessy (1999/2007). *The Cambridge History of Ancient China: From the Origins of Civilization to 221 BC*. Cambridge, U.K.: Cambridge University Press.

Mair, Victor H., tr. (1994), *Wandering on the Way: Early Taoist Tales and Parables of Chuang Tzu*, Bantam Books

Lutz, Antoine; Richard J. Davidson; *et al.* (2004). "Long-term meditators self-induce high-amplitude gamma synchrony during mental practice". *Proceedings of the National Academy of Sciences*

Chapter 7.

Rudolf Chorchia: Hypnose & Systemik, Lehrbuch, (2012)

Mascot, C. (2004). "Hypnotherapy: A complementary therapy with broad applications"

Barrett, Deirdre. "The Power of Hypnosis.". Psychology Today. Jan/Feb 2001

Astin, J.A.; Shapiro, S. L.; Eisenberg, D. M.; Forys, K. L. (2003). "Mind-body medicine: state of the science, implications for practice". *Journal of the American Board of Family Practitioners*

W. Barker and S. Burgwin (1948). "Brain Wave Patterns Accompanying Changes in Sleep and Wakefulness During Hypnosis". *Psychosomatic Medicine*

Kroger, William S. (1977) *Clinical and experimental hypnosis in medicine, dentistry, and psychology.* Lippincott, Philadelphia

Morgan J.D. (1993). *The Principles of Hypnotherapy.* Eildon Press

Asokananda: *Traditionelle Thai-Massage für Fortgeschrittene*. Bangkok, (1998)

Hubert; Patanant, Montien: *Lehrbuch der traditionellen Thai-Massagetherapie*. München Jena, (2007)

Wujastyk, D. (2003). *The Roots of Ayurveda: Selections from Sanskrit Medical Writings. Penguin Books.*

Mamtani, R.; Mamtani, R. (2005). "Ayurveda and Yoga in Cardiovascular Diseases". *Cardiology Review*

Subhose, V.; Srinivas, P.; Narayana, A. (2005). "Basic principles of pharmaceutical science in Ayurvĕda".

Kishor Patwardhan (2008). Concepts of Human Physiology in Ayurveda, in *Sowarigpa and Ayurveda*, Central Institute of Higher Tibetan Studies

Alice Burmeister with Tom Monte: The Touch of Healing; Energizing Body, Mind and Spirit with the Art of Jin Shin Jyutsu (1997)

A Nancy Recant Production (Video): Jin Shin Jyutsu^R: The Art of Living; A tribute to Mary Burmeister (2001)

Chapter 8.

Wile, Douglas (2007). "Taijiquan and Taoism from Religion to Martial Art and Martial Art to Religion"

Wang, C; Collet JP & Lau J (2004). "The effect of Tai Chi on health outcomes in patients with chronic conditions: a systematic review". *Archives of Internal Medicine*

Friedman, P. and G. Eisman (2005). *The Pilates Method of Physical and Mental Conditioning*. USA: Viking Studio

Flood, Gavin (1996), An Introduction to Hinduism, Cambridge University Press

J. A. Santucci, *An Outline of Vedic Literature* (1976).

Jan Gonda: *Die Religionen Indiens*. Bd. I: *Veda und älterer Hinduismus*. Kohlhammer, Stuttgart u.a. 2. A. (1978).

Chapter 9.

Galdston, I. (1960). *Human Nutrition Historic and Scientific*. New York: International Universities Press

Thiollet, J.-P. (2001). *Vitamines & minéraux*. Paris: Anagramme

Kendall Powell (2007 May 31). "The Two Faces of Fat"

Davis, B. and Melina, V. 2000. *Becoming Vegan.*

Rodrigo G, Carrera J, Jaramillo A (2007). "Evolutionary mechanisms of circadian clocks". *Central European Journal of Biology*

Art Martin, PhD.,N.D.: Your body is talking; Are You Listening?

K.Korotkov: Aura nad Conciousness: New Stage of Scientific Understanding

Chapters 10. - 14.

Cabot Sandra, M.D.: The Liver Cleansing Diet

Johnson Richard, M.D.: The Sugar Fix: The High Fructose Fallout that is Making You Fat and Sick

Myss Caroline: Anatomy of The Spirit (1966)

Wild Helmaring Doris: Think Thin, Be Thin: 101 Psyhological Way to Lose Weight (Broadway, 2006)

Oxford Vegetarian Study

Schweizerische Vereinigung für Vegetarismus

Key J. Timothy, Fraser, E. Gary et al.: Mortality in vegetarians and Nonvegetarians, American Journal of Clinical Nutrition 70, Nr.S. Sept 1

www.ingramcontent.com/pod-product-compliance
Lightning Source LLC
LaVergne TN
LVHW020658110826
845149LV00012B/2035

* 9 7 8 3 0 3 3 0 3 7 0 1 4 *